CONTROLLED
CHEATING

Also by Larry Goldberg

GOLDBERG'S DIET CATALOG
GOLDBERG'S PIZZA BOOK

CONTROLLED CHEATING

The Fats Goldberg
Take It Off, Keep It Off Diet Program

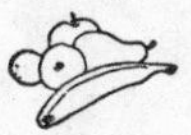

LARRY GOLDBERG

Doubleday & Company, Inc., Garden City, New York
1981

Library of Congress Cataloging in Publication Data

Goldberg, Larry.
Controlled cheating.

1. Reducing diets. 2. Reducing. I. Title.
RM222.2.G594 613.2′5
ISBN 0-385-17379-2 AACR2
Library of Congress Catalog Card Number: 80–2838

PRINTED IN THE UNITED STATES OF AMERICA
FIRST EDITION

For my folks

Sara and Art Goldberg, my sister Joc,
whose money I snitched as a kid so I could eat more and . . .

Goldberg's Market
3843 Agnes, Kansas City, Missouri
"Fancy Groceries and Meats, Free Delivery (me),
Call WA 0030"

ACKNOWLEDGMENTS

Rochelle Larkin, friend and writer, who said,
"Goldberg, write this book!"

Jody Greco, friend and nutritionist, who said,
"Goldberg, this will work!"

Lindy Hess, friend and editor, who said,
"Goldberg, do some work!"

Foreword

by Robert Bernstein, M.D.

This is a surprising diet book. In fact, it isn't really a diet book at all. I think that's fortunate, because over my years of practice it has become clear to me that diseases requiring dietary control are, practically speaking, untreatable. Hypertensive patients who previously ate little or no salt will suddenly crave pickles and pastrami as soon as their doctor bans them. All of my diabetic patients love sugar. And I suspect that even my children, who despise most vegetables, would binge on cauliflower and broccoli if I ordered them to avoid those foods. Treatment of obesity is the worst problem, because seemingly everything that tastes good is forbidden. Since prescribing diets invariably evokes a confrontation between the doctor and even the most reasonable patient, thereby rendering any future therapy hopeless, I rarely prescribe diets. Traditional diet books are more hopeless still, and most of them wind up on a shelf, collecting dust next to Shakespearean sonnets and Victorian novels.

If CONTROLLED CHEATING isn't a diet book, what is it? It's a testimonial to the successful method of Larry Goldberg, who, at forty-seven years of age, is half of his former body weight, despite constant exposure to his own pizza and all of the other temptations for sale on the streets of New York. Larry is one of the few people who has gone from 325 to 150 pounds—and kept the weight off for twenty-two years.

How can a man who hadn't been able to diet for a single day manage to keep his weight down for over two decades? The secret seems to be removal of guilt. Obese people have always been told that they shouldn't eat all sorts of foods—ever. Accordingly, as soon as they deviate from their diets, they feel like failures. And how have they learned to respond to failure? They eat even more, of course! But Larry was able to stay on his diet for two full weeks before his first day of "controlled cheating." Why? Because he knew that on selected days after that he would be able to eat to his heart's content without feeling guilty. Like Larry, I'm in my forties and I weigh 160 pounds. And I love to eat almost everything. I was never fat, but, like most "naturally thin" people, I watch my weight carefully. In fact, my secret is my own variation of controlled cheating. Over the years, I have eaten my share of "diet foods," but I have also eaten more than my share of goodies, including Goldberg's pizza.

Although the word "cheating" might suggest that you should feel guilty about eating, as you read this book you will find that the emphasis is on *controlled* cheating. The book is full of behavioral techniques that will enable you to maintain your diet despite temptation. Larry also tells you how to handle restaurants, travel, parties, and how to change your inappropriate eating habits. The book also has low-calorie recipes and a nutritious diet program. But, of equal importance, it tells you how to enjoy your cheating days to the fullest without losing control and how to maximize your pleasure on those days in a way that will carry you over the following diet days.

I also like Larry's emphasis on physical activity, since I have rarely seen a person lose a large amount of weight and maintain the loss without increasing his or her level of activity. Goldberg's formula is very sensible: lots of walking, incorporating physical activities into your daily life, and doing things that you enjoy.

There has never been a perfect book on weight control, and there most likely never will be. However, unless you require a special medical diet (for diabetes or hypertension, for example), Larry's overall program is consistent with the principles of good nutrition.

Will controlled cheating work for you? If you now eat very little and still have a weight problem, probably not. But, if you, like Fats Goldberg, eat large quantities and find it impossible to limit your food intake for long periods by other means, this may be the system for you. Go ahead and try it! You have nothing to lose but your fat . . .

Robert Bernstein, M.D.,
Medical Director, Weight-Control Unit,
St. Luke's-Roosevelt Hospital Center,
New York City

Contents

There is no love sincerer than the love of food.
—Bernard Shaw, *Man and Superman*

CONTROLLED
CHEATING

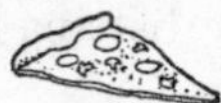

Bringing Up Fats

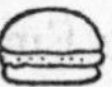

BREAKFAST: Two scrambled eggs, very soft; three buttermilk pancakes the size of hubcabs; four strips of crisp bacon; four golden-brown link sausages; six homemade biscuits with a quarter pound of butter and half a jar of Smucker's strawberry preserves; half a quart of whole homogenized milk (not that funny, anemic bluish-white stuff they call skim milk); two homemade cinnamon rolls.

MID-MORNING SNACK: Two of Kresge's chili dogs; giant foamy root beer.

LUNCH: Hot roast beef sandwich swimming in thick lumpy beige gravy; three slices of Butternut bread to lap up the gravy; a quarter of a Dutch apple pie, a la mode; two Cokes.

MID-AFTERNOON SNACK: One-half of a fresh banana cake with half a pint of chocolate ice cream.

DINNER: Three Winstead's Drive-In double cheeseburgers with everything; order of fries; chocolate Frosty Malt; fresh-lime Coke.

MOVIE SNACK: Box of hot buttered popcorn (extra butter, please); large Dr. Pepper; two Payday candy bars.

AFTER-MOVIE SNACK: A $1.69 Zarda Dairy banana split, no maraschino cherries.

LATE-NIGHT NOSH: Big slice of homemade cherry pie; sixteen ounces of Pepsi.

No, this is not what King Kong and Fay Wray ate on the way to the Empire State Building. This is what I ate in one typical day on a recent visit to my home town, Kansas City, Missouri.

In eight gorging days and nine gluttonous nights, I put on a fast eighteen pounds. Eighteen pounds in eight days is a little heartburning even for me, but when I came back to New York, I lost twelve of the eighteen pounds in three weeks. I do this twice a year. It's good for my soul, but, oh, my poor body.

You see, that's me in the photo—the fat, grinning Buddha with the large earlobes. Or rather, that was me, eighteen years ago, when I weighed an incredible 325 pounds. The slim matinee idol is me, too—last month when I slipped in at 150 pounds. I had lost a whole Goldberg. But the monster's ready to come back to life any time I slide back to my old gorging habits.

I am a foodaholic. I mainline Mallomars. I'm a Chunky junkie. Even the word "food" conjures up mouth-watering dreams of hot drippy pepperoni pizza, huge Cokes with crushed ice, crisp crinkly French fries so greasy my fingers are slick, and thick chocolate shakes with little lumps of vanilla ice cream still floating around.

Nothing used to get between me and food. When I was twenty-two and had just graduated from college, I had a complete physical, the first one of my life. After putting me through some horrible tests, the doctor took me into his office, shut the door, and announced that I had diabetes (of the latent variety—but quite real enough for me). My three double chins started to tremble; I was terrified. But, he said, I could control my diabetes through diet. I regained my composure, walked out the door, got in my car, and drove to Winstead's Drive-In—and ate three double cheeseburgers (everything except onions), two fresh-lime Cokes, and a chocolate Frosty Malt. When I was fat and got hungry, the angel of death could be sitting on my shoulder and I wouldn't miss a bite.

Very funny. Unfortunately for most fatties, it's the old story of laughing through the tears. And the world doesn't make it any easier. First of all, I have to eat every day to live. Even worse, when I walk down any street, I see and smell delicatessens, pizza stands, Baskin-Robbinses, and the hot pretzel pusher. Food is all around us.

And there is no way a food addict can get a non-fattening fix. I walked through my local supermarket and proved that, for two bucks, I could gobble either five pounds of bananas, or two big bags of potato chips, or one and a half pecan coffee cakes, or six Eskimo Pies, or nine Twinkies, or fifty-four Oreo Creme Sandwiches, or a jar of Skippy peanut butter, a jar of grape jelly, and a loaf of Wonder bread. But there are virtually no non-fattening snacks that I can buy and eat on the run. If I can't get—or don't want—foods like fruit or pickles, I have to chew my knuckles.

How did I get into this bind? When I was born, forty-seven years ago, to Sara and Art Goldberg of Kansas City, Missouri, I weighed seven pounds fourteen ounces. Sara, who weighs 140 pounds, is the Jelly Bean Queen of Kansas City. She still hangs around Woolworth's candy counter eating candy orange slices. Art weighed 150 pounds, never got hungry, and owned a food emporium called, not surprisingly, Goldberg's Market—"Fancy Groceries and Meats," with free delivery. (I was the free delivery.) Jocelyn, my sister, is five years older than me . . . and skinny. Lucky Joc.

Ma says I was a "chunky" baby and that I was eating everything in sight while I was still gurgling in her arms. In third grade I weighed 105 pounds. By sixth grade, I weighed a cool 200 pounds. When Ma would cook she'd make six pork chops;

one for each of them and three for me. I was so "chunky" I couldn't sit in a normal desk. Mrs. Burns, my teacher, had me sit in a straight chair on the side of the room.

My pediatrician once hauled me up on the table when I was a little fat kid and said, "Do you want to die in ten years?" I tipped in at 240 in the eighth grade. After I waddled to three doctors, they diagnosed my malady as a severe case of overeating. This is when the diets started. Every doctor would gaze at my stomach and give me a mimeographed sheet with sample diets for seven days. You know the kind: Breakfast was half an orange, a poached egg, a slice of dry toast, and half a glass of skim milk. Lunch and dinner were just as boring. I'd bring the diet home, diet through breakfast, and blow the whole deal at lunch.

My parents couldn't stop me from eating—no parents could. They'd have had to keep an eye on me twenty-four hours a day. If I couldn't eat at home or in the grocery store stockroom, I'd eat at neighbors', friends', strangers', or any place where I found a spare cashew.

Popping diet pills came during my freshman year at high school. It started with one pill a half hour before each meal, each pill a different color. I ran the whole diet pill string, from the worthless ones through the powerful Dexedrine spansules that made me giggle a lot. None worked for long. The minute I'd stop taking the pills, I'd start eating all over again. The only real difference in my life was that now I was terrified all the time, a perpetual hypochondriac.

High school was a lot of laughs. I bought a 1937 Oldsmobile that started leaning toward the left. Anyone who sat next to me automatically slid down the nylon seat cover to my side. That could have been exciting, except I had only two dates in high school. Both were with the same girl on consecutive New Year's Eves. Four friends and I were supposed to go out stag. But both times they got dates and fixed me up without telling me, until they surprised me on the big night. They knew I wouldn't have gone if I'd known. I was plenty mad and also plenty scared.

Actually, there was one other date in high school—the Sunday school confirmation dance. Everyone in the class had dates except me and Lucille Parelman. Poor Lucy was almost as fat as I was, so the Sunday school teacher arranged the fix up. That was one of the worst evenings, I'm sure, that either of us had spent in our entire lives. We just hung around the refreshment table the entire evening. The amounts we ate were about even, but I think she may have outdone me a little. We danced once. That was the first time I'd ever held a girl in my arms—also the first time I'd ever danced. But we were so big our extended arms could barely touch each other's sides. You should have seen us cha-cha.

My official weight when I graduated from high school and got my draft card was 265 pounds. Kansas City Junior College was next.

During my first year I sold ladies' shoes at a local Baker's Shoe Store and got my nickname of "Three Cases Goldberg." Selling a "case" in shoe peddling means selling $100 worth of shoes. For me, though, the name applied not to my sales, but to my size—300-pound Goldberg.

In college guys are supposed to become clothes-conscious, but I did all my Beau Brummell work at either Sears or the local army-navy store. They were the only places that could fit me. My costume never varied. First I wore Sears Roebuck's "Armored Crotch" boxer shorts—I could swear that was the brand name. They were reinforced between the legs because you know how fat boys chafe. Then I wore size 17½ white or blue oxford-cloth button-down shirts. I was a 300-pound sex bomb with saddle shoes.

When I moved on to the University of Missouri to study journalism, I pledged Zeta Beta Tau fraternity. There I went formal and switched to 48-inch-waist khakis instead of the overalls. I now weighed 305 pounds, and had managed to kiss one girl, once.

I always tried to take a shower alone in the fraternity house because I was embarrassed by my size. One day I happened to glance at my naked body after taking a shower. I noticed a string of little red scratches circling my tummy. Although I tried never to look at myself completely undressed, now that I had done so, panic set in. I ran to the doctor, who told me those red lines were stretch marks. That is, the skin couldn't hold the fat. He reassured me that they were harmless and that pregnant women get them all the time. But, I whimpered, I wasn't a pregnant woman. I was thoroughly depressed until I could get to a pint of butterscotch swirl ice cream.

Once during my first year, after I had eaten three complete lunches in one hour, I thought I had finally done it: I was going to die from overeating. Struggling over to the infirmary, I bared my soul to the doctor. I begged him for a diet. Being more accustomed to mononucleosis than to cases such as mine, he pushed his finger in my stomach, shook his head, told me to cool it on the groceries, and sent me home. He didn't realize he was dealing with an addict—and what an addict!

The worst night I ever spent during my fat years was in the fraternity house, two months before graduation. As usual, after my customary three-and-a-half-portion dinner, I started to watch TV or thumb through a book. And—again as usual—I started salivating around eight-thirty, waiting for the sandwich man who came around at ten o'clock. But that night he didn't show. By eleven-thirty I was in a state of panic. Everything was closed except for the highway cafés and the doughnut shop in downtown Columbia, and, to top it all off, it was snowing. I ran from room to room, sweating and screaming for someone to take me to eat. At last, Dave Goodman, God bless him, took pity on my crazed condition and drove me to the Broadway Donut Shop;

after a dozen hot glazed doughnuts and a quart of chocolate milk, I finally stopped twitching.

After I graduated from college in journalism, I had four jobs that first year. I counted Japanese thong sandals in bins, sold radio time for a rock station in Kansas City, went back to Columbia, Missouri, as a radio announcer (calling myself Fats Goldberg, the Sheik of Columbia), and was a television announcer, off camera of course. Finally I wound up in Chicago working for the Chicago *Tribune,* and it was there that I made a decision. I was tired of being fat. It was ugly and uncomfortable, the morning heartburn really hurt, and being fat was rapidly becoming a lot less funny than it had once seemed.

So on Monday, May 1, 1959, I awoke and rubbed my food-swollen eyes and said to myself, "Today's the day I'm going to start my diet." I'd said those words to myself almost every morning since the day I was born. But this was it. The last time I'd weighed myself was three or four months before when I'd found a freight and cattle scale. (Household scales, at least the ones I've seen, only go to 300 pounds.) I hopped on the freight scale, and when the needle started careening over 300 and wasn't slowing down, I leaped off. It had hit 325.

On the first day of the rest of my life, I literally rolled out of bed and took a Dexedrine spansule diet pill. After a breakfast of two scrambled eggs, an English muffin, and two cups of coffee, I decided there'd be no more diet pills for me. Either I was going to do this cold turkey, just me and my stomach, or I'd just keep eating until my navel popped out and I'd die, having lived a short fat life.

For lunch, I had to meet a car dealer to whom I was trying to sell ad space in the *Tribune,* and he wanted to go to a smorgasbord. What a way to start a diet! But I ate only a couple of pieces of roast beef and a few green beans. And for dinner I held myself to steak and cottage cheese.

The first three letters of diet, as was pointed out in something

I once read, are *die*. By my second day of dieting, I believed death would have been easier. I didn't think I could take dieting any longer. With no exaggeration, my whole body from my hair to my corns craved and demanded food. Still, I gritted my underused teeth and somehow stuck it out.

At 325 pounds, 190 was my goal, but it seemed to be a lifetime away. It took me twenty-five years to put that weight on and I wanted to take it off in three days. The second week I lost seventeen pounds. I didn't care if it was water or cheesecake, I was losing weight. This made me feel great. I was accomplishing something. I could feel it and I could see it when I got on the scale.

When I made that decision to diet, I had to make a total commitment to a new life-style. If I was going to lose weight, I had to stop eating. So when the hunger pains were making my stomach do the Charleston, I would think about Caterpillar tractors, joint sessions of Congress, Marilyn Monroe—anything except food.

Somewhere along the line, I read that the proper way to eat was to breakfast like a king, lunch like a prince, and dine like a pauper. I used that system for years and it works, though I've now developed Goldberg's variations on it, about which you will hear more later. At that time, I would get up in the morning, drink a glass of skim milk to get me rolling, then follow it with two eggs, toast, and coffee. Sometimes I'd throw in a little bacon or sausage. Lunch was a sandwich and a glass of skim milk. I always took the top piece of bread off and folded the two halves together. That way I saved the calories in a slice of bread. Dinner was meat of some kind, or chicken or turkey, with cottage cheese or tomato.

One of the hardest things for me to learn was how to add variety to my diet. I used to find a food that would let me lose weight and I'd eat so much of it I'd get to the point where I couldn't stand to look at it anymore. Fresh pineapple is one example. It was juicy, cold, and sweet, and it filled me up. But I ate so much leaves almost started growing out of my head. Boredom is a dangerous feeling when you're dieting.

Crawling up that slippery road of dieting, I could feel my poor vacant tummy getting weary of the struggle already. Shoot. And this was only after the first three weeks. Here I go again; the old diet elevator, the Overweight Otis, the Wagonload Westinghouse, up and down the scale; lose 10, put back 15.

After a fast start, I looked at the cloudy horizon and saw that nothing good to eat was in the forecast. I choked back a tear. I knew I had to try a different road without a map from any of the diet plans that hadn't worked before.

Then it hit me like a ton of warm glazed doughnuts—*Controlled Cheating*. I was going to pick one glorious day out of every week and eat anything in the world I wanted. Finally, there was a light at the end of the tunnel, a diet tunnel that was only six days long. Even old weak Fatberg could stay on a mean, dumb diet for six days when there was manna and everything else from heaven on the seventh.

Controlled Cheating was a simple plan and a life plan I maybe could live with for the rest of my days and be happy *and* skinny.

The first Cheating Day was a Sunday and brought caloric joy to my deprived body. I had pecan pancakes with lots of butter and syrup, pepperoni pizza, hot popcorn, two Pepsis, and a bagel with cream cheese.

Ah, but there was a cigar butt in the banana cream pie. Could I go back on the diet after that one happy Cheating Day? The next morning I hopped on the scale. Help me God, four pounds gained. My eyes glazed over like doughnuts with panic and pain. Okay, this was the supreme test. I set my quivering jaw and started back into the mine shaft. After all, it was only six stinky Diet Days back to heavenly Sunday.

During that week, I lost the four pounds I had picked up, plus an additional three. Happy days were here again and Sunday was coming.

Looking back over all those dumb diets I could never stay on, I realized this was *the* problem. A person can't look down that long road of life and never see another hot fudge sundae. *Controlled Cheating* was the answer. Strict dieting with nutritious foods for six days, with one day off for gluttonous behavior.

My experience of the past twenty skinny years convinced me that Controlled Cheating is a weight-loss-and-maintenance plan that can work for any man, woman, or child, regardless of how much or how little they want to lose, and to *maintain that ideal weight.*

My overall goal was to lose 135 of my 325 pounds, but being weak and not knowing how long I could last without a food reward, I set intermediate goals. The first goal was to weigh 265 pounds when I went on vacation to Kansas City after three months of dieting. When I walked in the back door of my house, Ma was peeling potatoes. She looked up and said, "Yes?" For a second, she hadn't even recognized her bouncing baby boy. I was thrilled.

Everywhere, in Chicago and Kansas City, people would notice the difference immediately. My size 52-long suits were getting very baggy. I woke up without heartburn. Everyone was tremendously encouraging and, when they got me alone, would ask how I did it. The management at the Chicago *Tribune* became more interested in my career. I was taken off probation on the company's major medical policy. I developed a new self-confidence and outlook on everything, including my social life.

Demon temptations were always around: pungent-smelling fast-food joints, or dinner in a restaurant or someone's house. But I learned how to cope by saying No, unless it was Sunday.

Pain was my constant companion—the physical pain of being hungry and the psychological pain of deprivation. I had to change my life-style to one that wasn't centered around food.

And I did it. In one year I lost 135 pounds.

When I weighed 190 pounds, I went into the pizza biz. I figured that if I couldn't eat it, at least I could become a pizza voyeur, selling and smelling the best and one of the most nutritious foods in the world. A son-of-a-gun-a mozzarella miracle happened. *New York* magazine had a pizza contest and Goldberg's Pizzeria was voted the best in the Big Apple.

There I was, at the age of thirty-four, crouched in front of two 650-degree ovens schlepping pizzas. It was like working the night shift at a steel mill open hearth in Gary, Indiana. My Health-O-Meter scale started to go down again. Terrific. Now twelve years later, I'm down to a constant 150 and as lean as a cougar.

It wasn't only sweating that peeled off the last forty pounds. I became an expert in losing weight, especially on my own personal system. Diet and nutrition books are like fried chicken to me. I can't get enough, but, after more than twenty years, the more I read, see, and talk, the more I'm convinced there is no fast, easy, and painless way to lose weight permanently. Dieting is a job, but, as with a job, I discovered I can have days off. That's the beauty of Controlled Cheating and why it works.

The usual history of the dieter is like that of a convict. After getting out of the prison of their fat, they regress and go back behind bars. What I want you to do is melt those nasty fat bars down *permanently*. That's what we're going to do right here.

With this system I developed, which I think of as Goldberg Oasis Method of Weight Loss and Maintenance, I figured I was slim enough to increase my Controlled Cheating to *two* days a week. I switched gears.

Now I ate everything my heart desired on Monday, storing up those delicious flavors and smells like a camel. I went back on the diet Tuesday and Wednesday. Thursday, I had another eating orgy to carry me through the lean days of Friday, Saturday, and Sunday. On a Monday or Thursday, I might add on five pounds. But I took off those hot pounds on the following Diet Days. I had to have those controlled binge days to look forward to—each a blessed oasis in the middle of that dry diet desert.

I doubled my pleasure and fun by that extra binge day a

week. Two days instead of one looked better than the numbers on a refund check from the I.R.S.

Controlled Cheating works. But it demands discipline.

Let's you and I sit down and have a serious talk.

Once you pick your Controlled Cheating Day or Days, those days cannot be changed.

I don't care if Christmas falls on a Saturday and your Cheating Day is Sunday or you are invited to dinner at Julia Child's or you're going home to Mom's apple pie and warm corn bread with sweet butter or that dynamite woman you've been panting to take out just said yes to dinner, you MUST stick to your plan.

We all have fourteen million reasons to go back to stuffing our mouths. There will always be excuses your tummy will broadcast to your brain to be filled up. You cannot change your Cheating Day for every hot excuse that comes along. Before you can say, "Big Mac," you'll be back gorging every day. Buck up, set your jaw, and dream of your coming Diet Oasis, because as you become lighter, so will the burden of dieting. Here's a new wrinkle I just developed recently.

Woe is me. Getting off TWA Flight #86 from Kansas City in September 1979, I was sad. I had just finished seven straight days of outstanding eating and now I had to go back to my knife and fork prison.

Hey, I thought, maybe I could change my Controlled Cheating diet plan a little now. After all, on May 1, 1979, I had celebrated my twentieth anniversary of being a successful dieter. Here I was, forty-five years old, in excellent health, and slim for the last half of my life.

What if I cheated every third day? Diet two, binge one. This would give me flexibility, too. Suppose my Cheating Day was Tuesday but I had a hot date on Wednesday. I could postpone the eating day to Wednesday. For the first time in my dieting life I had some flexibility. I didn't have to be as rigid.

Plus it would add sixteen more Cheating Days annually to my life. Sixteen more days of blissful eating.

My new plan has worked. It's been almost a year and I still weigh 150 pounds. It's great, but remember, I only got to my two days on, one day off after years of successful, rigid Controlled Cheating. Of course, if you have less to lose than I did (325 to 150, kids), you may get to this stage much faster than I did.

After a time of cheating once a week, and then twice, it's easy to stay with this plan for the rest of your life *and never gain weight again.*

But now, back to some more basics.

All right, Goldberg, Mr. Hot Shot Dieter, what do YOU eat on your dieting days?

Hold still, Controlled Cheater, here goes: Since I work nights, I get up at nine in the morning in time to roll over and watch Phil Donahue and do a little yoga exercising. I force myself to get on my exercise bicycle and peddle a hard fifteen minutes while reading *People* magazine. After that I eat four tablespoons of raw bran, washing them down with four glasses of water. Then after my shower, a glass of orange juice.

I leave my spacious two-and-a-half-room apartment about noon and walk a mile and a half to the Gaiety Delicatessen. There I dine on slices of turkey, or tuna fish, or chicken salad, or chopped liver, plus a toasted buttered bagel and a glass of skim milk.

After that sumptuous repast, I walk another couple of miles and usually stop for a glass of fresh squeezed orange juice at about three or four in the afternoon. I go to work where I'll gnaw on an orange, banana, or apple. An hour or two later, I'll have some Grape Nuts or hot-air popcorn (no butter or oil) with skim milk. About seven o'clock I might munch a salad or drink some fresh vegetable juices and for a nightcap an orange or apple.

This menu can vary as to time and foods eaten but I always eat a balanced diet. As you can see, I eat about six little meals all through the day. This way I always have something to look forward to. I eat no red meat on my Diet Days. And I drink about ten or twelve glasses of water a day, too. People can always tell when Goldberg dances down the street: They hear the sounds of sloshing.

There are a few rules I've set up for myself on my Diet Days.

1. Eating a balanced diet.

2. Eating slowly, putting my fork DOWN after every bite and not picking the fork up again until after I swallow. Before I lost weight, I ate like a runaway windmill—one whirling, continuous circular motion from the plate to my mouth and back again as fast as I could.

3. Be flexible. Add a variety of low-calorie foods to the diet. Boredom in eating the same foods every day is a dangerous emotion for a fatty.

4. I pray a lot.

Still, by eleven o'clock, I'm against the wall with hunger. Sometimes it gets so bad that I can't wait to brush my teeth, so I can at least get the taste of Crest toothpaste.

I also dream of food. (I have this recurring dream of bakeries . . .) Sometimes I wake up feeling sorry for myself. But I have twenty-five years of outstanding eating behind me, and I remind myself that I probably ate more in those twenty-five years than a normal person would eat in a lifetime. I feel better when I look at it that way.

For years, I saw myself as a trim Burt Lancaster or a rugged Gary Cooper. Right now I'm svelte, but I'll never be rugged. And as for shoulders, I didn't come equipped with any. My formal exercise is limited to my stationary bicycle and to a little yoga—shoulder stands (possible even on my meager shoulders) to save my hair. I also do lots of walking—a fast three or four miles a day on the hard New York concrete. This keeps me in pretty good shape, and keeps my podiatrist happy.

There you have it—the way I live and diet. The diet path I've chosen works for me. My fat outlook on life has changed to thin. I am finally a "normal" person, though "normality" was a shock at first.

As a fat man I was safe. That big wall of fat protected me. While other kids were going through the trials of puberty and dating, I escaped by eating my way through adolescence. No wonder I didn't go through puberty until I was thirty-one. No one could get close to me, literally or figuratively. Kidding and teasing were important to keep people away. But now that I'm thin, I don't have to hide behind my fat. I'm more honest about how I feel. And this gives me something I never had—self-confidence. I have become more relaxed and self-assured. Other people look at me with respect, which is a totally new sensation.

After going through the disciplines of dieting, I feel there is nothing I can't handle. In my B.C.C. (Before Controlled Cheating) days, I couldn't call a woman for a date without the phone sliding out of my sweaty hand. Not that I became a swaggering boulevardier or a Robert Redford overnight, but my social life *is* a social life, a full and happy one, not a bunch of excuses and alibis hiding behind a wall of fat.

There are also other big bonuses. I can go into Brooks Brothers without the salesman giggling, snorting, and hiding behind the crew-neck sweaters. I can sleep on my stomach without having a stomach ache in the morning. I've stopped gnawing my fingernails. I can wear LaCoste knit shirts without looking like two St. Bernards in a bag fighting to get out. I have a hundred times more energy and require three hours less sleep. Ties don't have to be extra long to fit around my 17½-inch neck. I can tie my shoes without crossing my legs. I can sit in a movie theater seat straight and not on my side. People will sit next to me on the bus. I don't perspire as much. Women look at me admiringly on the street. Clothes don't wear out as fast. I can see and feel my bones. I can get in and out of the smallest cars. I even bought a Volkswagen. I have stopped snoring. Sometimes someone says I am too thin and should eat more. I can be the last one on a crowded elevator.

AND if I live even one minute longer because I lost weight, it was all worth it.

YOU'D BETTER READ THIS

I'm taking one whole page—and pages cost much money—to tell you something. No, more than tell you—beseech you, command you. And you'd better damn well do what I tell you!

Before you do anything in this book:

GO TO YOUR DOCTOR AND DISCUSS THE DIET WITH HIM!

I'm going to repeat this throughout the book until you're sick of it, but it's your health I'm worried about.

P.S. I do not work for the American Medical Association.

Born to Lose

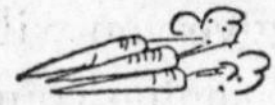

This chapter is basically a Texaco roadmap for the rest of the book, with stops along the way while I point out short cuts, roadblocks, and detours to make the diet trip easier for you. There's a lot of misinformation out there that could get you stuck in the mud, and there are a lot of directions you might not know.

WHO'S WILL POWER

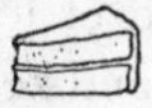

Hey Will Power, hey Willie Power, come out, come out wherever you are. You're not there? How come? Everyone says you have to have something called "will power" to lose and keep off weight. The big problem is that there is no such thing. That's right—if there was, I would have found it. For forty-seven years,

I've been looking for that son of a gun in every diet book and under every piece of apple pie. If I had waited to find will power, I would never have lost 175 pounds.

Will power is a cop out. It's the most overused, dumb expression ever invented, and I should know. I conned myself for twenty-five years with that usual excuse: "I don't have any will power." There is no magic for losing and keeping weight off. No blinding ray of light will shoot down from the parting fat clouds to give you will power.

Imagine yourself sitting at the kitchen table. In front of you is a big soup bowl of creamy soft French vanilla ice cream, topped with homemade hot fudge, which is making little brown and white rivers, and chunks of roasted almonds like little rowboats rushing down the rapids. That bowl is screaming for you to grab a tablespoon out of the drawer and bless your mouth with indescribable joy—and no will power is going to hold your quivering shoulders and shout a great big NO! in your ear.

GOLDBERG POWER

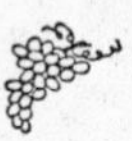

If I, weak Fats Goldberg, can lose 175 pounds and keep it off for twenty-two years, then you, frustrated person, or anyone else who ever gnawed on a head of iceberg lettuce trying to lose a few ounces, can lose weight and keep it off. I guarantee it.

Let's you and I pull up a couple of ice cream chairs and talk about Goldberg Power. I'm not Superman or even Darth Vader. What I am is a fat man disguised as a thin man. (I don't have the shoulders to be Superman and I used to need about four times the space of a phone booth just to put on my boxer shorts.)

What's Goldberg Power? Very simply it's DO IT! DO IT! DO IT!

Aren't you getting tired of reading diet books, fantasizing about being thin and good-looking with enough energy to roller disco all night and run a five-mile race in the morning?

For me, twenty-two years ago, and now for you, too, the time for talking is over. Now is the time to act. First, there is no such thing as a perfect time for you to start dieting. The time to start is now.

Smarts, discipline, laughs, thinness, and everything else you'll ever have or want are dancing inside that beautiful body of yours. No one but YOU can make you lose weight and keep it off. The only way to release that tremendous power you have is to start tapping your great ocean of inner resources. Once your strengths start gushing to the surface, a Texas oil well will look like a drop in the bucket.

Losing weight and keeping it off is a difficult business. At different times for the rest of your Controlled Cheating life, every ounce of guts you can muster will help you *not* to eat that Twinkie.

I'm going to be with you every step of the way because I've already gone down that Yellow Mozzarella Brick Road to the Emerald City. What all this boils down to is whether or not you're going to eat that pepperoni pizza when you shouldn't.

The first step in using your power is to set a realistic goal of how much total weight you want to lose. After you've done that, put the number away in the freezer of your mind so it won't spoil.

HOW TO FIGURE YOUR GOAL WEIGHT

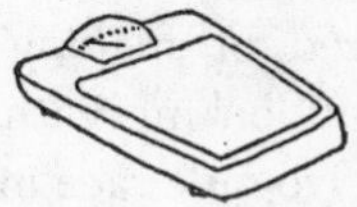

This is the area of dieting most open for individual interpretation. I can tell you how and what to eat, what not to eat, and describe a series of exercises to get you where you want to be, but only you and your doctor can decide what that shape or size is.

I think that goal is something most overweight folks already know about themselves. I don't believe it's necessary to go to the lists printed by the insurance companies of ideal weights, except perhaps as a general guide. We all know at what weight or size we felt most comfortable and looked our best. For women, this may translate into being the size they were when they got out of school or when they got married. For men, it may be the "fighting weight" they were when they played ball. Or it could be the weight we were at any time during the years before we started adding pounds.

Whatever you decide to lose, you must stick to that number as your Goal Weight. It will determine where you are and when your Cheating Days will be increased. Naturally, if you reach your goal and feel you would look even better a few pounds less, you can make that your new goal and diet down to it, sticking to your routine until you get there.

GOLDBERG'S FIVE-POUNDER

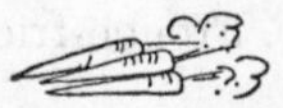

No, this doesn't come from under a Golden Arch with pickles, onions, mustard, and ketchup. This is my system for setting your Goal Weight, getting to it, and sticking to it. You know what your ideal weight is, or what you want it to be.

Once you've set your Goal Weight, think of it as divided into Five-Pound Bites. When you've chewed away the first Five-Pounder, go for another Five-Pounder and then all the weight down. If you're more than twenty-five pounds overweight, your ultimate goal may seem impossible, but taking it in five-pound bites will give you reachable, intermediate successes that will spur you on to the next Five-Pounder. Soon all the Fives you subtract will add up to your true goal!

You might say, "Hey, Goldberg, I have to lose fifty-five pounds. Five measly pounds is nothing."

If you don't think five pounds is much weight, I want you to take the Goldberg's Safeway Supermarket Schlep Test. Here's how:

Go into your local grocery store and pick up a five-pound bag of potatoes and hoist it over your head. That's the weight you have just taken off your poor sagging bones. You might get some funny looks from blue-haired ladies thumping watermelons, but just smile triumphantly.

After you lose another five, go back and lift ten pounds over your head. The same ladies will probably still be there. If they call the manager, run to the detergent department and hide. Keep testing with every five-pound loss until you think you might get a hernia.

Everything you do for yourself takes time. It took a long time to put on that fat and there is no way you're going to lose it overnight. That's why Controlled Cheating works. You'll only have to diet for two short weeks at the start; then every week after that, you'll be able to eat as much as you want of whatever you want for a whole day. French-fried everything, here I come!

PICKING THE DAY TO START YOUR CONTROLLED CHEATING

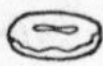

Monday is the best day to start your diet. How come? I started my diet on a Monday, twenty-two years ago, and I'm generous enough to want to give you every advantage I had.

Everyone else starts their diets on Mondays, so you'll have lots of grumpy company. Of course, the obvious reason is that everybody hogs it up on the weekends and feels guilty, as they are bursting out of their tight jeans on Monday morning.

The weekend is the toughest time for us weight losers. Everyone is off work, running to the beach, shopping, or just lying around the house trying to remember some area of the refrigerator they haven't already explored. Social events are mostly on weekends and who can resist dinner at the home of a great cook or the wedding of your cousin's daughter's niece where the caterer is a sugar sadist?

When you start on a Monday, there are five full days to lose some weight and build your mighty resolve before the critical weekend when you want to stick your whole head in a gallon of rum raisin ice cream and can't.

Anyway Mondays are rotten! Work begins again, the weekend's over, it always rains on Monday, bills come on Monday, folks are normally in bad moods, and the only good show on television is Monday Night Football.

When you start dieting on Monday, it will be only one of a

hundred other miserable things you're doing and you won't even notice you're eating a wilted lettuce leaf.

CHEATING BEFORE YOU DIET

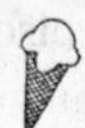

Okay, you're ready. You've made the biggie, that rock-hard decision. This coming Monday, regardless of what you have to do or how you feel, is D (Diet) Day. Feel better already? You bet. No more horsing around, no more waiting until after Groundhog Day, or after that Yankee-Red Sox doubleheader so that you can stuff down the juicy hot dogs with horseradish mustard and cold foamy beer.

From now until THE Monday, eat what you want, but in moderation. Don't make those first two weeks any harder than they are already. This is the time, just before your diet starts, to start eating the way a thin person eats. After all, that's what you're going to be from now on. Don't eat like a loco grizzly bear who has to put on an extra layer of suet to keep warm through the winter. Or like a condemned man getting that final meal on earth before Pat O'Brien, as the priest, comes in to walk you down that last mile.

That's the joy of Controlled Cheating, a new, thin life, where you don't have to give up anything, where all the foods you love the most will be ready and waiting for you every single week.

Some of the most helpful parts of my program are not usually mentioned in diet books. But dieting is a permanent part of my life. I want it to sing along in harmony with other things that are important to me. I couldn't diet successfully without a sense of humor, plenty of quick smiles and—surprise—the power of prayer, plus a lot of other fun stuff.

GOLDBERG GETS YOU THROUGH

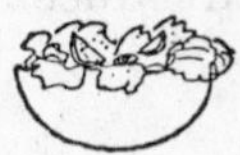

SMILE

Smile: It's one of the best exercises and you don't need Adidas.
Smile: It stretches certain muscles and will make you glow down to your toes.
Smile: As you picture yourself a thin person, completely in control of your mouth and life, no longer a prisoner fighting to get out of a bag of nacho-flavored Doritos.
Smile: While you think about the new slim you.
Smile: At your self-confidence, sense of accomplishment, party-going, and the tight T-shirts you can wear.
Smile: Know you are wonderful already and that losing weight and keeping it off will only improve a good life.
Smile: To yourself and know deep down nothing can stop you from reaching your goal. (You may even giggle out loud once in a while.)
Smile: Your body will laugh with relief from getting rid of that excess fat.

THE LIGHT TOUCH

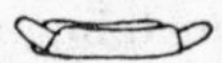

Relax and Take It Easy

Sit back, take off your saddle shoes, prop your feet up with the holes in the socks, loosen your belt (you might have to anyway), scratch wherever it itches, and relax. You're about to start on a long tour because I want you to live to be 120.

Controlled Cheating is a lifetime tap dance. Because it is a plan that lasts the rest of your life, being twitchy, tense, nervous, irritable, and an all 'round nudge won't work. Besides, folks won't want to hang out with you. You must learn to relax and take it easy. DO NOT take yourself too seriously.

None of us are perfect and you're going to make mistakes. And you're going to make errors that will cost you rotten, filthy pounds. I still make mistakes, plenty of them. At times, I feel I can play my body like a 150-pound Stradivarius strumming the Sabre Dance. But on any Diet Day, I can eat all the right foods, get plenty of exercise, do everything right, and *pow,* eat something stupid that I think is low-calorie and, of course, it isn't.

Hopping on the scale the next morning, I scream with terror. That dumb needle didn't move down, and even worse, I slapped on a pound.

Over the years, I've learned to say over and over in the relaxer section of my brain, which is right next to the panic button, relax, relax, RELAX. The more you take it easy and relax, the more energy you'll have for dieting.

I also cool it by singing, whistling, and talking to myself. Sometimes I even do it out loud, which is fine in New York because most folks talk to themselves out loud anyway—and nobody notices.

LIKE

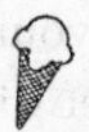

I like "like." Love is a nice word, but it sort of falls out of your mouth. Say love and your jaw drops open, your tongue looks like a soggy washcloth, and love dribbles out. Like has a fresh, crisp sound, and you can hardly say it without smiling.

I like myself. I'm my own best pal. When I started dieting, I didn't like myself. Folks wrote me off as another fat guy who couldn't keep his hand out of the groceries. My self-esteem was lower than the last drop of Heinz ketchup in the bottle.

My first big break came when the Chicago *Tribune* gave me a job in 1958. There I was, over 325 big ones, one suit (which I couldn't button), a 1951 pea-green Pontiac, a bag of stale bagels, and six warm Pepsis. But the Chicago *Tribune* liked me. That made me feel terrific. They had confidence and accepted me for what I was. That made me *want* to be better.

I didn't understand all this in 1958, but I started dieting. I was plain tired of being fat, so I began losing weight. Looking in the mirror at my vanishing body and buttoning my pants with ease, I began to like myself more.

Then other people noticed and started yelling about how good I looked. A few took me aside and asked how I was doing it. My diet plan was just starting to take shape—like me. The more I lost, the better I felt about myself. The better I felt about myself, the more my family and friends gave me a pat on the buns. The more patting, the less buns.

The whole thing is a big wondrous circle that you can jump into anytime, too. Look inside yourself. Look outside yourself. You're going to like what you see.

The First Hurrah

Everyone, including you, needs a cheering section: a warm body you can talk to when your stomach feels as empty as the Grand Canyon, when you get discouraged, depressed, and want to nuke the whole diet idea.

Depend on your family, friends, or just one good pal. You can call them any time of the day or night. Get everything out on the table. Maybe shed a tear or two. I do. They'll give you an encouraging word, I promise.

HUGGIN' AND KISSIN'

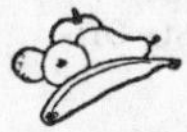

Hugging and kissing are the best exercises mentally and physically for any and all occasions. The three best things in the world are sex, food, and air conditioning—and not necessarily in that order.

Sex is the number-one, best, all-time cure for the diet blues. As Dr. Theodore Rubin, the famous formerly fat psychiatrist, says, "Next time you're hungry, reach for your mate instead of your plate."

What else can I say about huggin' and kissin' that you haven't already thought of and probably practice better than I do? Only the following:

This is a public service announcement that will eliminate confusion and be of great help in using sex to lose pounds. Here are the actual calories used per hour during sex. Really, this is no joke.

*Calories Used Per Hour During Sex**

Weight (In Pounds)	110 lbs.	150 lbs.	200 lbs.
	CALORIES USED	CALORIES USED	CALORIES USED
Foreplay	80	100	115
Intercourse			
a. Aggressor	235	300	350
b. Submissor	105	135	155

* *From: The Exerciser's Handbook* by Charles Kuntzleman, Ph.D., National YMCA Consultant, David McKay Company, Inc., Publishers; $5.95. Copyright © 1978.

These calories refer to calories used per hour. If the sex act lasts fifteen minutes simply divide by four; twenty minutes by three; thirty minutes by two; and so on.

Personal Observation from Fats Goldberg

This chart clearly fails to take into consideration wild foreplay and intercourse in a hot room on an August afternoon in The Acme Motel on Route 66 in Braceville, Illinois. I personally have lost three to five pounds in such activity besides curling my hair and clearing my sinuses.

MIND GAMES

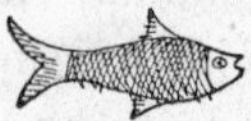

Flicks, Fun, and Fantasy are all mental sports to help take your mind off food. In my hunger-crazed nights, I have imagined some of the following movies on the silver screen of my mind. See these and then try to direct some of your own. You might win an Academy Award.

The Following Motion Pictures Have Been Rated G: Suitable for Audiences of All Ages

Anything Goes . . . For Dieters Starring Clint Fatwood, Candice Calorie, Pinky Levis, and Larry Fatberg as The Couch

The life story of Sigmund Freudfood done in rhyming couplets and Portuguese animated cartoons. A heartwarming saga of how Siggy psyched up dieters of all ages to use anything their minds can conjure to stick to their diets, at only $75 for forty minutes. Exciting violent action scenes of dieters going to movies, popcornless; leaning against a Greyhound Bus in Aubrey, Kansas, meditating; lurking around Arthur Treacher's, sniffing grease.

Title Song Sung by Kate Smith

Pumping Imagination Starring Arnold SneakSnicker, 1959 Mr. Sara Lee Strawberry Cheesecake; Sally Fieldgoal, Jockey Schwartz, Wendy Hot and Juicy, and featuring Lars Goldbarge as The Pump

A Western with a message. How stretching your imagination will make it happy, strong, and without stretch marks. There is also a tender love scene between Sally and Arnold where she tells him she'll follow him anywhere if he promises her a thin life and swears to take off his six-shooter in bed.

Costumes by Fruit of the Loom

The Gizzard of Odds Judy Garland O'Lakes, Bert Lard, Jack Honey, Ray Bulger, Margaret Hamburger as the Wicked Witch, Billie Burp as the Good Witch, and introducing "Shep" Goldbark as Tushie the Dog

A stupendous musical extravaganza directed by Vincent Manicotti which tells the electrifying saga of how, on the silver screen of your mind, you can picture yourself slim by whirling around with a fork in a tornado made of low-fat cottage cheese, celery, and Perrier water. The climax is you playing quarterback for the Dallas Cowboys or walking down the runway in Atlantic City as Tushie bark-sings "Miss America" to you. As the credits roll you are crowned a twinkly star in the Paradise of Thinness.

These motion pictures will be opening in my mind. Open some in yours, too. They're great.

PRAYER

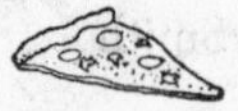

Yeah, I pray. Prayer makes me feel good. Being Jewish (oh, you knew already?), most of my organized prayer has been in synagogues. But I've done some heavy-duty praying in Catholic, Baptist, Congregational, you name it, churches.

My personal belief is that God is everywhere and has a great sense of humor. If I want to talk to Him (or Her), I can be eating a juicy sirloin and buttery hash browns, kissing a lady, running for the subway, white knuckled on an airplane, or anywhere. I do plenty of praying on airplanes. Deep down, I'm an evangelist, a thin evangelist, preaching the joys of a normal, skinny life. (I'll deliver my sermon on the Mounds at the end of the book.)

Prayer can work for you. It's the best and cheapest do-it-yourself mental health. You'll be amazed at the number of hunger pains God can take away.

I pray almost every night after Johnny Carson and before I go to sleep. I thank God for the day, for keeping me lean, and keeping my family and friends safe. Then I give God all my problems, ask for a good day tomorrow, roll over, and dream of chocolate doughnuts.

THE FIRST DAY

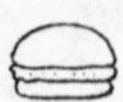

The clock radio clicks on, playing "Junk Food Junkie," jolting you back from a yummy dream of climbing up a mountain of fresh ripe strawberries on a shortcake ladder while you're carrying a bag of whipped cream.

Sleep catches you with all your defenses down. At no time in your dieting life are you more vulnerable. Rub the sleep from your eyes, slap a smile on your face (see "Goldberg Gets You Through," above), and leap out of bed. Today is THE DAY.

You scream, "Oh God, no! It's Monday and I have to start my Controlled Cheating Diet Program that some guy named Goldberg says has worked for him for over twenty years and will work for me. If he's such a hot shot dieter, let him do it for me. I'll start tomorrow—maybe."

Right there, right at that instant, stop that thought and replace it with a positive proclamation starting your diet today. That's NOW, not tomorrow, or next week. This is called Positively Waking Up. Like everyone else, I have negative, dumb thoughts when I wake up. I've discovered that if I can substitute good, positive vibrations shooting through my brain for the first fifteen minutes, I have the rest of the day made.

You can use this system, too. It takes practice, but soon it will come automatically. What a difference it will make in your life. Think about the food hangovers, volcano-hot heartburn, and the Milky Way-stained shirts you'll never have again.

When you've got your mind giggling, tap dance into the bathroom and, with plenty of sweet toothpaste, give your teeth the workout of their lives. While you're riding the Crest, start thinking about fourteen days from now and the good eats you're going to choose for your Controlled Cheating Day. See, right away you can look forward to a pot of gold, or at least pasta, at the end of the rainbow.

I want you to look forward to your diet meals, too. We all know how much fun eating is. Make your breakfast, lunch, dinner, and snacks big, happy events. You might even blow up a few balloons. Plus, if you eat very slooooooowly, the fun of eating will go on and on.

Don't start feeling sorry for yourself, ever. Especially not on this crucial first day. So you don't get to eat a hunk of creamy cheesecake. So what! You've only got to wait for a couple of weeks and you can have nine pieces of creamy cheesecake—plus a glass of cream, if you want.

I know, I know, you're so hungry you're about to start licking the plaster off the walls. Hey, I'm right with you all the way. After twenty-two years, I still get as hungry on Non-Cheating Days as I did the first day I started. YOU CAN DO IT. If I, Fats Goldberg, foodaholic, human garbage can, and all-around weak person, can do it, you sure can. Why? Because we can look at that beautiful horizon and eyeball your gorgeous Controlled Cheating Day.

Schlep this book along with you on the first day and every day for the next two weeks. *Really* learn what you can and cannot eat, and, just as important, the portion sizes. Make notes in it, draw funny faces, put your home room number in the front. Read it while you're eating. If you're lucky, maybe a few crumbs will fall in the pages. Later in the day you can lick your finger, pick up the crumbs, and have an evening snack.

Your first Diet Day is about over. Congratulations, you soon-to-be-thin person. I know you've stuck to the diet. *Hooray!* Only thirteen more days until Broadway, your first Cheating Day.

Tomorrow morning you'll get up, hop on the scale, and maybe see some results from today. Don't get twitchy if there is no movement on the scale right away. We lose weight in stair steps, not in a perfect slide. That stupid needle might not move right away, especially at the beginning, and then *pow,* you'll drop a whole load of pounds all at once—and you'll keep on dropping.

As I tuck you in, and you snuggle down for an indigestion-free sleep, before I tiptoe out, I must scream that under no circumstances are you to take any diet pills or any over-the-counter appetite depressants or diet aids. Save your money for an extra dessert on a Cheating Day; it'll do you more good.

THE FOURTEEN LONGEST DAYS OF YOUR LIFE

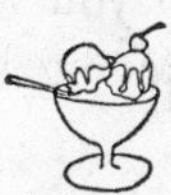

Congrats, you've gotten through the most awful day and night of your Controlled Cheating life. Now what's thirteen more Diet Days to a diet professional like you? But wait, don't break your arm patting yourself on the back. (It's all right to give yourself a few hugs, though.)

I know you can sail through the weekdays of dieting like a swift breeze. After all, you've got your career, or there's the fun of housework, or whatever you do Monday through Friday. The sticker is the weekend. You must double your determination on Saturday and Sunday. When you get down to it, there are only four measly days you have to worry about. Keeping busy is the answer. The devil finds Twinkies for idle hands.

Here are some Weekend Wonders that I've used:

1. Make a big list of activities for each day: Clean out the garage; play golf, tennis, stick ball, or all three; go shopping (stay out of supermarkets unless accompanied by a friend or relative with a strong pair of handcuffs); or go to a museum. I especially like museums because there are no refreshment stands and you can meet a fancy, smart person.

2. Stuff your ice box with big bowls of cut up vegetables and fruits, such as carrots, celery, tomatoes, cauliflower, and other crunchies. On Diet Days I like foods that require heavy chewing and make plenty of noise. You can fake yourself out that you're having huge meals, plus filling your tummy with good nutrition at the same time.

3. If you are going out to dinner or a hot party, eat some of those low-calorie foods before leaving home. They'll take the edge off your appetite. Then you won't leap into the middle of the goody table or start gnawing your way through the bread and butter basket.

4. Drinking alcoholic beverages is forbidden during the first fourteen days. Stick to plain tap water, the chic sparkling water with a spritz of lime, coffee and tea (no sugar or cream, please), or sugar-free soda with lots of ice.

5. Think about your Controlled Cheating Day and what you're going to eat.

6. Go see *Grease, Sugar Babies,* or a Meatloaf concert.

SLIM PICKIN'S

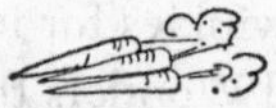

In the next chapter, my nutritional consultant, Ms. Jody Greco, and I are going to raise the curtain on the specific weight-loss program for Controlled Cheating: Fats Goldberg's Take It Off, Keep It Off Diet Program, for light-eating, Non-Cheating Days.

Here's the menu:

1. We want you to start your nutritional education with some basic information. For example, did you know that you have to consume 3,500 excess calories to put on a pound of weight? And that you have to cut out 3,500 calories to take off that pound? These and other amazing facts will make you the life . . . and death of any party.

2. The diet itself is based on the report of the 1977 United States Senate Select Committee on Nutrition and Human Needs.

You can't get any better nutritional information than that. Finally, you're getting something from Washington besides hot air.

3. You will be given fourteen days of diet menus for men and women. There can be no messing around for these first fourteen days. You must eat the exact amounts and the exact specific foods. After the first fourteen days, there will be hundreds of substitute and free foods, foods that you can eat all you want of and enough variety so you won't get bored.

4. You'll find exciting demonstrations on calorie-saving cooking and many diet recipes. Included will be my very own recipe for diet pizza. There's no dough or crust.

5. Rhumba over to the phone, take your chocolate-covered finger and dial your beloved doctor. Make an appointment for a complete checkup. Before you start any weight-loss program, YOU MUST SEE YOUR DOCTOR FIRST. The next time you see him, he may not recognize you!

ROW, ROW YOUR BOAT

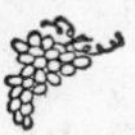

Everybody up! Don't sit there. Time to start moving that body. To lose a size, E-X-E-R-C-I-S-E! Physical movement, along with diet, is the only way to lose weight and keep it off. I know you're famished and there's enough room in there to play the 1982 Super Bowl, but your best bet is to go for a schlep or ride your bicycle.

A little workout will flush the gook out of your head and use up some calories, too. Say you're a 150-pounder and you've been watching television for an hour, you've burned 100 calories. But take a long walk for an hour and you'll use up 210 calories. That 110-calorie difference is a slice of white bread. If you move a little faster for that hour, you can knock off 300 calories.

Your heart, lungs, ears, toes, and everything else will thank you, too. Exercise is a critical part of Controlled Cheating. In a later chapter, I'll give you all my exercises including walking, stationary bicycling, running, rope skipping, and running up and down seven flights of stairs five or six times a day.

I'm the laziest guy I know. I only work out about an hour a day and I've never been in better shape. One little trick I use on my Cheating Days is to exercise more. Then I can eat an extra butterscotch praline ice cream cone.

A big shot nutritionist a long time ago told me that all this diet business can be summed up in one sentence: "To lose weight and keep it off, you must eat less and exercise more." And that's the truth.

CONTROLLED CHEATING

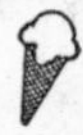

Those two words should be tattooed on my tummy. They should be etched in mozzarella on my headstone.

HERE LIES
FATS GOLDBERG
1934–2054
I OWE IT ALL TO CONTROLLED CHEATING
REST IN PIZZA

Without Controlled Cheating, I probably would have gone to that Big Burger King in the sky many years ago. This system, program, plan, or whatever, which I developed is the only way

I've lost a whole Goldberg and kept him away for twenty-two years.

Controlled Cheating eliminates the problems that have caused dieters to fail throughout history. Ivan couldn't diet; he was Terrible. Catherine practiced Controlled Cheating and she was Great.

Here's why:

1. Controlled Cheating is healthy. It's a variation of the system which medical authorities consider the proper way to lose weight and keep it off.

2. Controlled Cheating is guilt-free because it's planned and controlled.

3. Controlled Cheating is fun because you plan your own Cheating Day and eat whatever YOU want.

4. Controlled Cheating proves that there is no "magic" to keeping slim, just plain hard facts.

5. Controlled Cheating releases the tight band from around your head of thinking you have to be on a diet *every* day of your life.

6. Controlled Cheating will change your body, your health, your life.

Hold on, we'll go through the whole program in the next chapter.

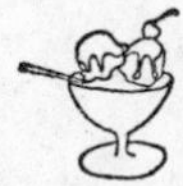

Take My Diet...Please

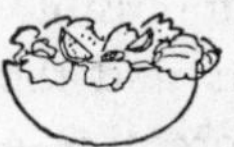

Before we begin this all-important diet and nutrition chapter, I want to introduce my nutritional consultant, Ms. Jody Greco. Jody not only helped me formulate the 14-Day Diet, but she compiled the nutrition information, and has read every fat word in this book. She even made notes while running in marathons. (Just yesterday she ran a quick twenty-one miles.)

Ms. Greco, will you please stand on your sore corns and meet the gang?

Jody has a Masters Degree in Public Health Nutrition from Columbia University and is also a Registered Dietician. She is currently employed by the federal government as a Public Health Nutritionist with the National Health Service. Ms. Big Time.

Thank you. You can sit down now.

WHAT'S SO NEAT ABOUT NUTRITION?

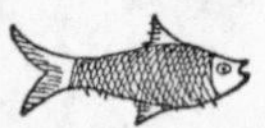

Nutrition is the connection between food and health. Proper nutrition means getting the right nutrients, in the right amounts, to insure your health and well-being. Without the right foods this is impossible. Too many diets, especially the so-called "crash" diets and those that depend primarily on one particular food, ignore this all-important principle. That's one of the reasons these diets inevitably fail. The dieter may lose weight, especially at the beginning, but the body soon cries out for the nutrients it is not getting and old eating habits return—generally with a vengeance!

No matter how important it is to any of us to be slim, it just doesn't make sense to lose weight and sacrifice your health. Most people diet to look good, and looking good always includes the glow, muscle tone, vitality, and energy of a healthy person.

That's why I've researched the food plan for your dieting, Non-Controlled Days so carefully. I don't just want you skinny, like *me;* I want you healthy, like me, *too!*

WHAT ARE CALORIES?

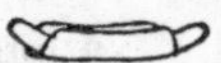

Calories are simply a measure of energy. As you probably remember from high school physics, energy can neither be created nor destroyed.

Your body is an incredibly efficient machine at saving calories. As you get older, your beautiful body requires even less calories to maintain its weight. So, when you give your body more calories than it requires, it stores the excess calories as fat.

All foods contain both nutrients and calories. It takes 3,500 calories to put on a pound of fat and you have to cut 3,500 calories from your intake to lose that pound of fat.

HOW MANY CALORIES YOU NEED PER DAY

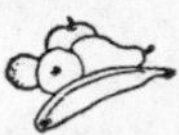

If your weight is about average, weigh yourself and multiply by 15. This will give you the amount of calories you need to maintain your present weight. For example, if you weigh 150 pounds, you multiply that 150 pounds by 15, and find that you have to eat 2,200 calories every day to stay at 150 pounds.

Suppose you *want* to weigh 125 pounds. Multiply 125 by 15 and that gives you the amount of calories, 1,900, you need per day to get down to your Goal Weight. You are taking in an excess of 300 calories per day.

If you want to lose one pound of fat a week, you must cut 500 calories from your intake per day. Multiplied by seven days, that gives you the total of 3,500 calories that equals one pound of fat loss.

FOOD

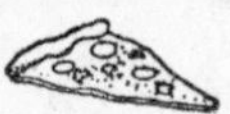

We get calories from four food sources: carbohydrates, proteins, fats, and alcohol.

Carbohydrates

Carbohydrates are starches and sugars. Carbohydrates have four calories per gram.

Proteins

Proteins have four calories per gram.

Fats

Fats, both saturated and unsaturated, have nine calories per gram.

Alcohol

Alcohol has seven calories per gram.

Most foods are a combination of carbohydrates, protein, and fat as well as vitamins, minerals, and fiber.

A lot of the foods folks think of as high-protein, like meats, cheeses, nuts, etc., are often very high in fat, too. And foods that people think of as high in carbohydrates, like doughnuts, crackers, and pie, are actually high in fat, also.

THE FIVE BASIC FOOD GROUPS

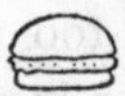

Most of the foods that are good for us fall into one of the five basic food categories. Eating from *each* of these five basic groups every day should give you all of the vitamins, minerals, and fibers needed for good nutrition. All are necessary for maintaining good health. The diet that you will follow on your Non-Cheating Days is formulated from these basic groups.

Fruits and Vegetables

All the foods that fall into this category are obvious. As these foods are best for you in their natural state, you should eat as many raw fruits and vegetables as possible.

This fruit and vegetable group provides you with all sorts of good vitamins, minerals, and fiber.

If a vegetable requires cooking to be edible, try steaming or cooking it for as short a time as possible using only a little water.

Nature has been incredibly generous in providing such a terrific variety of fruits and vegetables, something for every taste, need, and occasion, and your choices on the diet should reflect this. Eat at least one deep-yellow or dark-green leafy vegetable every day.

For freshness and flavor, buy your fruits and veggies in season whenever possible. Out-of-season fruits are extremely costly, and you're paying for their air fare to your neighborhood. (And since they've aged during the trip, they have less nutritional value.)

Very briefly here are some good sources of vitamin C: citrus fruits, cantaloupe, strawberries, cabbage, tomatoes, broccoli, peppers, and leafy vegetables.

Some good sources of vitamin A are dark-green leafy vegetables, carrots, and fruits, such as peaches, apricots, and mangoes.

Be careful about drinking too much fruit juice. Many fruit juices are high in calories. For instance, an eight-ounce glass of unsweetened orange juice has 120 calories but a medium orange has only sixty-five calories. If you choose the orange juice, you'll be missing all the valuable chewy, fibrous pulp from the orange. You'll also miss the thrill of having your fingers smell like orange for the rest of the day.

Breads and Cereals

From this group we get vitamins, minerals, and protein. It includes the starchy vegetables, such as corn, lima beans, peas, potatoes, and dried beans.

Dairy

This very important group includes milk and milk products, such as whole, skim, and low-fat milk, buttermilk, yogurt, and all cheeses. However, be sure that the dairy products you buy are made from skim and low-fat milk.

These foods provide calcium (the major source of this vital nutrient for most Americans), protein, and several vitamins, including important amounts of vitamins A and D when the product is labeled as fortified.

Meat, Fish, and Poultry

This is another varied food group. Members of this group are found on land, sea, and in the air. Besides the more familiar parts such as chops, breasts, and fillets, we also consume organ meats (liver, kidneys, and brains). In addition to meat, fish and seafood, and poultry, this group also includes eggs and contains many very valuable nutrients, primarily protein. Important minerals are found in this group and here, as with fruits and vegetables, our diet provides you with meals ranging widely among these foods. However, like the dairy group, many of the foods in this group contain cholesterol. All meats contain cholesterol, but the highest concentration is found in egg yolks and organ meats.

Fats and Oils

Choose a polyunsaturated fat, such as a corn oil or safflower oil, rather than a solid-type shortening such as lard, butter, and some margarines. Basically any fat that is liquid at room temperature is unsaturated. If you buy margarine, be sure to get a margarine that is sold in a "tub" instead of a hard stick. Remember to use only three teaspoons of any type of fat per day.

There you have it. I could go on describing food groups until my eyeballs and yours glaze over. All that's necessary here is that you understand why I have selected the diet that follows.

EATING LESS BUT DOING IT MORE OFTEN

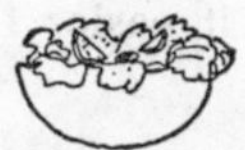

If you looked ahead to the 14-Day Diet, you noticed that each day allows for six separate table times. Three of those are the conventional basic meals, and three are allowed official snack times. Shortening the time between meals will help you consume less food more easily. There will no longer be the interminable hours stretching between breakfast and lunch and lunch and dinner, and perhaps, worst of all, the long dark night after dinner before the next day's breakfast. It's easier to be satisfied with a curtailed diet meal knowing that there's some relief and indulgence in a snack before the next meal.

Many doctors and nutritionists like the idea of six small meals a day even for the non-dieter, because it's easier for the body to digest food in smaller quantities. Three square meals a day, eaten according to the clock, is a convention that has no real basis in human needs. It's most probably a product of the increasing conformity that has been going on for centuries.

That's why I like the idea of having six mini-meals, by saving one fruit from breakfast, lunch, and dinner to make a mid-morning, afternoon, or evening snack, perhaps with a permitted beverage, or snacking on those highly nutritious vegetables on the "eat freely" list, or saving any of the other items on the menu to make six small meals instead of three large ones.

DIET SHOPPING FOR DIET EATING

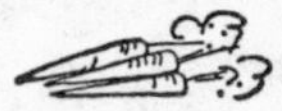

Proper shopping for the dieter is really a matter of following a few simple rules. But, as in most things, simple is good. Shopping correctly will make it easier to stay on your diet. Here's what to do:

1. Shop once a week for everything you need for your six dieting days. The less exposure to food, of course, the better. If you can't do it all in one day, at least shop as seldom as possible. By no means allow yourself the agony of facing 10,000 supermarket items every dieting day of your life.

2. Always shop *only* with a list. Your prepared shopping list is your lance in the supermarket wars, your primary defense against the archenemies of overspending and overeating. Naturally, your list will only include the items on your diet.

3. Never shop when you're hungry. That is to say, *really* hungry. On this diet, you're never going to feel overstuffed or possibly even totally full. You will almost always have a *little* hunger with you. But the time to shop is after you've had one of your main meals and the pangs have died down.

4. Don't take more money than you think you'll need. When temptation slips in, the money subtracts and the pounds add up. High-calorie foods are usually high-priced. Prepared foods, with a lot of ingredients and chemical additives, have no place on this diet and the counters and showcases that contain them should be avoided.

THE BASIC DIET

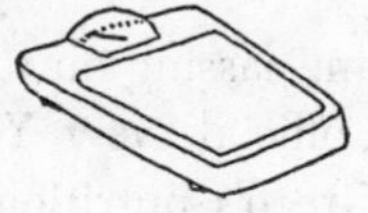

Are you ready? This is the hard part: the way you're going to eat on the days when you're not Controlled Cheating. It's not easy, but remember two important points:

1. When you have slogged through the first fourteen days of NO cheating dieting, you're going to have lost enough weight to put you right on the royal road to your goal. What you accomplish after these first two weeks is going to be easier and possibly more self-satisfying than anything you've ever done before.

You'll have proven you have the power to control your own life, the way you look, and the way you feel. This is more than most people manage to accomplish in a lifetime—and you've done it in two weeks! You're a *champion!*

This sense of accomplishment will spill right over into the rest of your life and make you deal with everything in a more effective way. Why? Because you'll know that your ability to succeed is much greater than you thought it was. Because your weight loss isn't something imagined, it's real. Because it isn't something that's been handed to you or that you read in a book. You've done it, and it's yours.

2. Coming at the end of the Famished Fortnight is something we've almost forgotten about as we've prepared you for the diet. That is, of course, your *first Controlled Cheating Day*—the delight at the end of the tunnel. Remember that after that first two-week blitz, you'll have a Controlled Cheating Day every week. Then three-quarters of the way to your Goal Weight, there will be two full days every week until you reach your own brand of perfection, at which time cheating will come every third day.

Okay, let's go.

The first basic diet I am passing on to you is our 14-Day Plan, which is based on the official New York City Department of Health Diet and Jody Greco's nutritional knowledge. The New York City Department of Health Diet is also here and it was formulated, tested, and used by hundreds of thousands of people and is the basis for almost every successful diet program in the country. Our program is especially for you but refer to the New York Health Diet for substitutions.

You may consider New York a great place to visit, but even if you wouldn't want to live here, you won't find a better-balanced, more nutritious, low-calorie diet anywhere. And you don't have to pay New York taxes or anything else to get it! In fact, the only requirement is the purchase, if you don't already have one, of a handy-dandy little kitchen scale that gives weight in ounces up to one pound. These are cheap and available anywhere. Once you have your scale, you're ready.

After you look over the 14-Day Diet Plan, you'll find the second diet program. This one is my baby, the one I actually used to lose 135 pounds in one year. Study both before you decide which one you want to follow. And, remember to consult your doctor. Check page 64 for "Other Foods to Eat Daily."

THE 14-DAY DIET PROGRAM

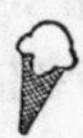

Day One

When Goldberg proposed this new diet
An overweight gal said, "I'll try it."
So she bought this book
And found what to cook–
"One potato–boil it–don't fry it!"

BREAKFAST

1 medium orange
2 ounces low-fat cottage cheese
1 slice whole-wheat bread
Coffee or tea

LUNCH

2 ounces lean hamburger, broiled
1 hard roll
Celery and carrot sticks
¼ pound grapes
Coffee, tea, or club soda

DINNER

Clam broth
4 ounces fillet of sole, broiled
Steamed broccoli
1 medium boiled potato
Romaine lettuce salad
1 peach
Coffee, tea, or club soda

Day Two

Day Two is where you'll find me.
Not to eat you don't have to remind me,
'Cause I'm getting slimmer,
Thinner and trimmer,
And my behind is closer behind me.

BREAKFAST

½ cantaloupe
¾ cup ready-to-eat unsweetened cereal with 1 tablespoon wheat germ
Coffee or tea

LUNCH

2 slices grilled cheese on rye with lettuce and tomato
½ grapefruit
Coffee, tea, or club soda

DINNER

1 cup tomato juice
4 ounces roasted veal
Spinach and mushroom salad
1 medium baked potato
½ cup fresh berries
Coffee, tea, or club soda

Day Three

Now we're at Day the Third,
Where chewing can barely be heard.
Just keep on pickin'
That four ounces of chicken.
You're eating (and just like) a bird.

BREAKFAST

1 cup tomato juice
1 ounce Cheddar cheese toasted on 1 slice of pumpernickel bread
Coffee or tea

LUNCH

Clam broth
3 to 4 ounces sardines in tomato sauce
1 hard roll
Cucumber and green pepper slices
1 apple
Coffee, tea, or club soda

DINNER

4 ounces chicken baked with herbs (take off the skin!)
Steamed zucchini
1 small ear of corn
Sliced tomatoes
½ cup unsweetened pineapple
Coffee, tea, or club soda

Day Four

The fourth day you get your great wish,
But only if it was for fish.
Don't sneer at your flounder,
He'd look a lot sounder
If he weren't so alone in that dish.

BREAKFAST

½ grapefruit
1 poached egg
1 English muffin, toasted
Coffee or tea

LUNCH

Chicken broth
2 ounces sliced turkey on 2 slices of rye bread
Pickles
Lettuce and tomatoes
1 pear
Coffee, tea, or club soda

DINNER

½ glass of vegetable juice
4 ounces flounder, broiled
Asparagus spears
Chicory salad with ½ cup diced beets
½ cup lima beans
2 small peaches
Coffee, tea, or club soda

Day Five

On the fifth day you see at a glance
It's easier to fit into your pants.
Soon your derrières
Will be smaller than Cher's
And your waistlines won't look like Lou Grant's.

BREAKFAST

½ glass prune juice
¾ cup unsweetened cold cereal with ½ cup skim milk
Coffee or tea

LUNCH

Consommé
4 ounces pot cheese
2 slices whole-wheat bread
Watercress salad
½ honeydew melon
Coffee, tea, or club soda

DINNER

4 ounces baked liver with onions
½ cup carrots
½ cup brown rice
1 tangerine
Coffee, tea, or club soda

Day Six

You've come all the way to Day Six;
You don't need that old food fix.
Your shape's getting smaller,
You even feel taller,
Like you could be playing for the Knicks.

BREAKFAST

8 ounces tomato juice
1 ounce Swiss cheese
1 slice toast
Coffee or tea

LUNCH

Chicken broth
2 ounces sliced chicken on a roll with mustard
Bibb lettuce and tomato salad
1 pear
Coffee, tea, or club soda

DINNER

½ cup of spaghetti with a sauce made of 4 ounces lean beef, ½ cup tomato puree, simmered with oregano, basil, and parsley
Escarole salad
Orange slices
Coffee, tea, or club soda

Day Seven

Here we are at Day Seven.
That means we're halfway to heaven.
But forget about manna,
Just enjoy your banana—
Even Moses got only unleaven.

BREAKFAST

½ cup grapefruit juice
½ cup oatmeal with 1 teaspoon of raisins, dash of cinnamon, and ½ cup skim milk
Coffee or tea

LUNCH

2 ounces water-packed tuna on 2 slices whole-wheat bread with sliced tomatoes
2 or 3 plums
Coffee, tea, or club soda

DINNER

4 ounces baked turkey breast
½ cup carrots and peas
Collard greens
1 small banana
Coffee, tea, or club soda

Day Eight

It's all downhill at Day Eight.
You're looking and feeling just great.
No candy, no pies,
So who'll criticize
'Cause you're licking the crumbs off your plate?

BREAKFAST

½ cantaloupe filled with 2 ounces low-fat cottage cheese, sprinkled with 1 tablespoon wheat germ and a dash of cinnamon
Coffee or tea

LUNCH

2 slices of lean roast beef on 2 slices of rye bread with lettuce, mustard, and pickle
1 orange
Coffee, tea, or club soda

DINNER

4 ounces haddock, baked with onion and red pepper rings
½ cup carrots
½ cup rice
Tomato salad
½ honeydew melon
Coffee, tea, or club soda

Day Nine

This day is like your Ninth Inning,
No wonder you're happy and grinning.
You've reached your dream,
You've made the "team,"
And what's more important, you're winning!

BREAKFAST

1 cup sliced strawberries with ½ cup plain yogurt
¾ cup cold unsweetened cereal
Coffee or tea

LUNCH

2 ounces water-packed salmon on a toasted English muffin
Chicory salad
Half round slice watermelon
Coffee, tea, or club soda

DINNER

4 ounces baked turkey
1 small sweet potato
Brussels sprouts
Lettuce and tomato salad
1 peach
Coffee, tea, or club soda

Day Ten

You look so terrific, you "10,"
What a difference between now and then!
The ladies are able
To think you're Clark Gable;
To the men you're Sophia Loren.

BREAKFAST

1 orange
1 egg
1 slice whole-wheat bread
Coffee or tea

LUNCH

2 ounces farmer cheese on toasted whole-wheat pita bread
Shredded red cabbage and carrot salad
½ honeydew melon
Coffee, tea, or club soda

DINNER

1 broiled pork chop
1 small ear of corn
Steamed broccoli
Mushroom and tomato salad
1 apple
Coffee, tea, or club soda

Day Eleven

This is the Eleventh Hour.
Of strength, you've become a tower.
You look sharp and lean
In your skin-tight jeans,
Thanks to less fats, less sugar, less flour!

BREAKFAST

4 ounces orange juice
2 ounces low-fat American cheese
1 slice whole-wheat toast
Coffee or tea

LUNCH

Tuna sandwich on cracked-wheat bread with lettuce and tomato
Tossed spinach and mushroom salad
½ cantaloupe
Coffee, tea, or club soda

DINNER

4 ounces hamburger, broiled with herbs
¾ cup baked winter squash
½ cup cauliflower
Mixed green salad
½ cup berries
Coffee, tea, or club soda

Day Twelve

Twelve so becomes you, my dear,
We make such a wonderful pair.
From using less Crisco
You're ready to disco—
And folks think that I'm Fred Astaire.

BREAKFAST

½ grapefruit
½ cup oatmeal with ½ cup skim milk
Coffee or tea

LUNCH

1 slice of Swiss cheese and 1 slice of lean ham on a hard roll with lettuce and tomato
Carrot sticks
½ cup unsweetened pineapple
Coffee, tea, or club soda

DINNER

4 ounces broiled bluefish
Spinach
1 small baked yam
Shredded cabbage salad
1 small banana
Coffee, tea, or club soda

Day Thirteen

Thirteen was considered unlucky
'Til you came along, oh so plucky.
No ice cream breaks,
Or big two-pound steaks,
Or chicken, fried from Kentucky.

BREAKFAST

1 tangerine
1 poached egg
1 slice whole-wheat toast
Coffee or tea

LUNCH

2 ounces broiled hamburger on a toasted English muffin
Brussels sprouts
¼ pound grapes
Coffee, tea, or club soda

DINNER

4 ounces chicken, baked with ½ cup artichoke hearts and lemon juice
½ cup rice
String beans
Escarole and cucumber salad
½ honeydew melon
Coffee, tea, or club soda

Day Fourteen

The two longest weeks of your life
Have ended without any strife.
To the food war you stagger
Not with gun or dagger,
Just a fork and a spoon and a knife!
Dig in!

BREAKFAST

½ cup unsweetened pineapple juice
¾ cup ready-to-eat unsweetened cereal with ½ cup skim milk
Coffee or tea

LUNCH

2 ounces pot cheese
1 plain toasted bagel
Tossed green salad with celery sticks and radishes
1 pear
Coffee, tea, or club soda

DINNER

4 ounces liver, broiled
Steamed asparagus
½ cup beets
1 small ear of corn
Half round slice watermelon
Coffee, tea, or club soda

RECIPE:

Broiled Liver-K-Bobs with onions, peppers, and tomatoes
Liver can be marinated in:
1 tablespoon soy sauce,
1 tablespoon lemon juice,
and ginger for ½ hour

Other Foods to Eat Daily

FAT:

3 servings daily
Use your fat allowance for cooking and in salad dressings. Remember that each *teaspoon* is about 25 to 30 calories.

1 teaspoon vegetable oil
or
1 teaspoon mayonnaise
or
2 teaspoons French dressing
or
1 teaspoon margarine

MILK:

Use your milk allowance in cereals and for a snack beverage in between meals or at bedtime.

2 cups (8 ounces each) skim milk
or
2 cups (8 ounces each) buttermilk
or
1 cup (8 ounces) evaporated skim milk
or
1 cup plain yogurt
or
⅔ cup non-fat dry milk solids

THE NEW YORK CITY HEALTH DEPARTMENT DIET*

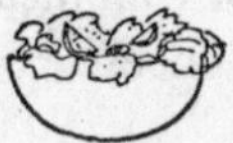

For Most Women and Small-Frame Men

Your 1,200-Calorie Menu Plan

BREAKFAST

High vitamin C fruit
  Choose ONE from Group 2
Protein Food–Choose ONE:
  2 ounces cottage or pot cheese
  1 ounce hard cheese
  2 ounces cooked or canned fish
  1 egg
  8-ounce cup skim milk
Bread or cereal, whole grain or enriched–Choose ONE:
  1 slice bread
  ¾ cup ready-to-eat cereal
  ½ cup cooked cereal
Coffee or tea

* Since New York City cannot afford to mail this diet out to each and every one of you, and since this diet has been used as the basis for so many others, I decided to reproduce it for you, courtesy of the Bureau of Nutrition of the New York City Department of Health.

LUNCH

Protein Food–Choose ONE:
- 2 ounces fish, poultry, or lean meat
- 4 ounces cottage or pot cheese
- 2 ounces hard cheese
- 1 egg
- 2 level tablespoons peanut butter

Bread–whole grain or enriched–2 slices
Vegetables–raw or cooked–except potato or substitute
Fruit–1 serving
Coffee or tea

DINNER

Protein Food–Choose ONE:
- 4 ounces cooked fish, poultry, or lean meat

Vegetables cooked and raw
- High vitamin A–Choose from Group 4
- Potato or substitute–Choose ONE from Group 5
- Other vegetables–you may eat freely

Fruit–1 serving
Coffee or tea

OTHER DAILY FOODS

Fat–Choose 3 from Group 6
Milk–2 cups (8 ounces each) skim or substitute from Group 7

For Most Men and Large-Frame Women *Your 1,600-Calorie Menu Plan*

BREAKFAST

High vitamin C fruit
  Choose ONE from Group 2
Protein Food–Choose ONE:
  2 ounces cottage or pot cheese
  1 ounce hard cheese
  2 ounces cooked or canned fish
  1 egg
  8-ounce cup skim milk
Bread or cereal, whole grain or enriched–Choose ONE:
  2 slices bread
  1½ cups ready-to-eat cereal
  1 cup cooked cereal
Coffee or tea

LUNCH

Protein Food–Choose ONE:
  2 ounces fish, poultry, or lean meat
  4 ounces cottage or pot cheese
  2 ounces hard cheese
  1 egg
  2 level tablespoons peanut butter
Bread–whole grain or enriched–2 slices
Vegetables–raw or cooked–except potato or substitute
Fruit–1 serving
Coffee or tea

DINNER

Protein Food–Choose ONE:
  6 ounces cooked fish, poultry, or lean meat
Vegetables–raw and cooked
  High vitamin A–Choose from Group 4
  Potato or substitute–Choose ONE from Group 5
  Other vegetables–you may eat freely
Fruit–1 serving
Coffee or tea

OTHER DAILY FOODS

Fat–Choose 6 from Group 6
Milk–2 cups (8 ounces each) skim or substitute from Group 7

Food Groups

1. Limit these protein foods
  Lean beef, pork, lamb to 1 pound per week total
  Eggs to 4 per week
  Hard cheese to 4 ounces per week

2. High vitamin C fruits (*no added sugar*)
  1 medium orange
  ½ medium cantaloupe
  1 cup strawberries
  ½ medium mango
  4 ounces orange or grapefruit juice
  ½ medium grapefruit
  1 large tangerine
  8 ounces tomato juice

3. Other fruits (*no added sugar*)
  1 medium apple or peach
  1 small banana or pear
  ¼ pound cherries or grapes
  ½ cup pineapple
  ½ cup berries
  2–3 apricots, prunes, or plums
  ½ round slice watermelon (1″ by 10″)
  ½ small honeydew melon
  2 tablespoons raisins

4. High vitamin A vegetables

Broccoli	Mustard greens,	Spinach
Carrots	Collards,	Watercress
Chicory	and other	Escarole
Pumpkin	leafy greens	
Winter squash		

5. Potato or substitute
   - 1 medium potato
   - 1 small sweet potato or yam
   - 1 small ear corn
   - ½ cup cooked rice, spaghetti, macaroni, grits, or noodles
   - ½ cup plantain, ñame, or yautía
   - ½ cup corn or green lima beans, peas
   - ½ cup cooked dry beans, peas, lentils
6. Fat
   - 1 teaspoon vegetable oil
   - 1 teaspoon mayonnaise
   - 2 teaspoons French dressing
   - 1 teaspoon margarine with liquid vegetable oil listed first on label of ingredients
7. Skim milk or substitute
   - 2 cups (8 ounces each) buttermilk
   - 1 cup (8 ounces) evaporated skim milk
   - ⅔ cup non-fat dry milk solids

YOU MAY DRINK

Coffee	Water	Bouillon
Tea	Club soda	Consommé

YOU MAY USE

Salt (but try not to)	Herbs	Lemon, Lime
Pepper	Spices	Vinegar
	Horseradish	

YOU MAY EAT FREELY

Asparagus
Green beans
Broccoli
Brussels sprouts
Carrots
Cauliflower
Celery
Chicory
Collards
Cucumber
Dandelion greens
Escarole
Kale
Lettuce
Mushrooms
Mustard greens
Parsley
Romaine lettuce
Spinach
Summer squash
Swiss chard
Tomato
Turnip greens
Watercress

YOU MAY NOT EAT OR DRINK

Bacon, fatty meats, sausage
Beer, liquor, wines
Butter, margarines other than described above
Cakes, cookies, crackers, doughnuts, pastries, pies
Candy, chocolates, nuts
Cream—sweet and sour, cream cheese, non-dairy cream substitutes
French-fried potatoes, potato chips
Pizza, popcorn, pretzels, and similar snack foods
Gelatin desserts
Puddings (sugar-sweetened)
Gravies and sauces
Honey, jams, jellies, sugar and syrup
Ice cream, ices, ice milk, sherbets
Milk, whole
Muffins, pancakes, waffles
Olives
Soda (sugar-sweetened)
Yogurt (fruit-flavored)

MORE FUN FOOD FACTS FROM FATS

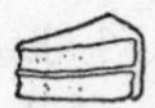

Instead of salt and pepper, try seasoning your food with a variety of herbs and spices. These perk up food flavors terrifically without adding calories. Some herbs have good nutritional value, too. If possible, grow your own or buy fresh rather than dried or processed. Meats, fish, and poultry can also be enhanced by herbs and spices. Experiment to find the combinations you like best.

Vegetables

Vegetables should be eaten raw whenever possible, and palatable. They may be cooked or steamed in water with no salt or oils added.

Fish

Fish should be baked, broiled, poached, boiled, barbecued, or steamed. Fry in oil only if you use part of the day's apportioned amount. Canned fish, such as tuna, should be packed in water, not oil.

Meat

Beef, lamb, and pork all contain fat. Limit these to one pound per week in total. Cut away all visible fat before cooking. Buy the leanest cuts available. Ask your butcher to grind your hamburger without any fat. Try making veal (which has very little fat) your main meat.

Meat should be broiled, baked, barbecued, or stewed with vegetables, or dry-fry on top of the stove in a non-stick fry pan.

Poultry

For the purposes of this diet, this means skinless chicken and turkey. Do not substitute duck or goose, which are both fatty fowls.

Poultry should be broiled, baked, poached, roasted, stewed, or boiled.

Eggs

Do not have more than four eggs or four ounces of hard cheese per week.

Eggs can be hard- or soft-boiled, poached or dry-fried in a non-stick pan, unless you use part of the daily oil allotted on the diet.

Hard-boiled eggs can be combined interestingly in salads with a variety of vegetables, as suggested in the diet, or you can create your own combinations.

Follow the instructions carefully, making sure to choose a wide range, especially from the fruit and vegetable groups, to add variety to your meals and insure your vitamin and mineral input.

Look at the list headed, "You May Not Eat or Drink," and every Cheating Day throw a copy of it out the window and yell Yippee.

MY OWN PERSONAL DIET OR HOW I LOST 135 POUNDS IN 12 MONTHS

I cannot look you straight in your chocolate-brown eyes and tell you that I lost all my weight on the 14-Day Diet Program included in this chapter.

Jody Greco and I developed the 14-Day Program especially for you from the very latest nutritional information available.

In 1959, when I started my own weight-loss program, there was no Jody Greco running around Kansas City.

But I was enough of a professional dieter to work out my own low-calorie balanced diet plan. My basic goal was simply to cut down the amount of calories I ate.

My diet is a more severe cutting back. I offer it to you as an alternative because I know how it worked for me. I want to share everything I know with you and, in this instance, give you a choice. If you want to diet my way, you'll find it very simple, because I offer fewer choices and less decisions for you to make.

Take a look at both diets and figure out which is best for you and your life-style. Maybe after a few months of getting used to Controlled Cheating, you can take the best of each program. That doesn't mean you combine the two and eat everything on both diets. You can't fool me.

Fats Goldberg's Controlled Cheating

This is the Fats Goldberg story,
He was the only mountain in Missouri
To curb his overeating
He created Controlled Cheating
Now he's nothing but skin, bones, and glory.

Breakfast #1

1. BOWL OF CEREAL

Choose a packaged whole grain cereal, either hot or cold. Eyeball all the ingredients on the package. If it includes sugar or salt, make sure they are low on the list of ingredients. Pour on just enough skim milk to cover the cereal to keep it crunchy. If you like to scuba dive with your spoon to find the cereal nuggets through a skim milk Lake Michigan, then be sure you wear goggles.

Grape Nuts are one of my all-time, anytime favorite foods. When you eat a bowl of Grape Nuts, the noise of the crunching, popping, and chewing in your head will make it seem like the Chicago Philharmonic moved in. With Grape Nuts, you know you've eaten something.

2. FRESH FRUITS

You can eat as much fruit as you like, either on the cereal, in the middle, or on the bottom depending on your mood. I love sliced bananas on my cereal. They float on top like little yellow rafts. If you're independent then eat fruits independently of the cereal. You can assert yourself.

3. DRINKS

Coffee or tea or ONE glass of skim milk optional

I once read that you should breakfast like a king, lunch like a prince, and dine like a pauper. This pat little saying has always made a lot of sense to me since I love a big breakfast or brunch. Also, we're coming out of an eight-hour sleeping fast and need food to stoke the furnace of our bodies. But not everyone feels that way about breakfast.

Let's say you're a queen and not a king and you can't stand the sight of breakfast. Then you must make your own personal adjustments. You don't have to eat as much as I've indicated. Feel free to eliminate one, some, or even all of the breakfast items or eat them later in the day, if you prefer.

Always remember, if you don't feel like eating, DON'T EAT! That's the most important point.

OR! OR! OR!

Breakfast #2 (only twice a week)

1. EGGS

You can have two eggs poached, soft- or hard-boiled, fried or scrambled. You egg experts who like your gold and white beauties fried or scrambled, try to make them in a non-stick pan. If not, use a teeny, tiny drop of butter or margarine. I love my eggs scrambled soft and runny so that I almost need a spoon to get every last morsel.

2. BREAD

ONE toasted bagel *OR* English muffin *OR* two slices of rye *OR* whole-wheat toast. Try to eat all breads dry. If you can't stand bread without butter or margarine, then use a teeny, tiny drop. Always buy whole grain breads. My biggest thrill with this breakfast is to lap up the eggs with the toast. Oh boy!

3. DRINKS

Coffee, tea, or *ONE* glass of skim milk optional

I ate basically this same breakfast, of ten to fourteen eggs per week, for many years, because I could look forward to a big breakfast. Man, how I love eggs and a bagel or English muffin.

My egg breakfasts were dynamite until my doctor discovered that my cholesterol was soaring to the moon, thanks mainly to those golden egg yolks which I soaked up with my bagel.

After I became the Cholesterol King, I cut Breakfast #2 down to twice a week. You should only eat Breakfast #2 twice a week, too. You've got to limit any eggs in your total diet to four per week.

By the way, cholesterol is saturated fats which are also found in most sweets, red meat, and whole milk dairy products. Many health honchos feel that too much cholesterol can be harmful.

Lunch

1. SANDWICH

That's *ONE* sandwich of turkey, chicken, or very lean roast beef. Make sure you pull the fatty skin off the turkey and chicken. Try to stay away from turkey or chicken roll. They're loaded with salt and all sorts of funny chemicals.

Whip the top slices of bread off each half and slap the two remaining halves together. You're only eating one slice of bread and you have a sandwich so thick it could spring your jaw out of joint. Use only whole grain breads.

Smear on mustard, if you want, but no ketchup (loaded with sugar) or high fat dressings such as mayo or Russian.

2. SIDE DISHES

Eat a lot of fresh fruits and raw vegetables. My favorites are crunchy carrots and celery, soft ripe bananas with the brown spots all over and zipper skins, juicy frigid melons, hard crispy apples, home-grown tomatoes (not those tasteless hothouse numbers), ice-cold pears, and navel oranges that leave your hands sticky.

3. DRINKS

Coffee, tea, or diet soda with plenty of ice and a lemon squeeze for pucker

Dinner

1. MAIN DISH

Chicken, pull the skin off before you cook it, baby. That's where all the fat hides. You can roast, broast, broil, or boil it: *OR* turkey, again yank the skin and throw it out the window: *OR* big hunk of fish, no butter, margarine, or other fats added. You can use tuna, but make sure the tuna is packed in water: *OR* small lean steak, broiled with all visible fattening fat removed: *OR* small lean hamburger pattie made with ground chuck or round steak, broiled. Ask the nice butcher to grind it special for you with no fat added.

2. SIDE DISHES

One plain old baked potato in the skin with no butter or margarine. Eat the skin too. It takes a while to get used to eating the skin but keep on gnawing *OR* a cup of brown rice *OR* a cup of peas (frozen or fresh, not canned) *OR* a cup of cooked dried beans *PLUS* crispy salad with low-cal or no dressing *PLUS* your favorite fresh fruits and raw vegetables.

3. DRINKS

Coffee, tea, diet soda, or fresh vegetable juices

Portion Sizes

There are very few portion sizes included on my personal diet. I really didn't even think about portion sizes when I started. What I did know is that if I ate small portions, I'd consume less calories and lose weight. If you want to weigh your food, great. If you don't, use your common sense.

Hunger

Only eat when you're hungry. When you feel full, STOP! You don't have to join the "Clean Plate Club."

Salt and Pepper

I never add salt or pepper and I don't think you should either. You're going to get all the salt you need in the prepared foods you eat. Ma Goldberg never had a salt or pepper shaker on the table. (I think she was afraid I'd eat the shakers.)

Water

Boy, do I love water. It's neat. Water is the only magic elixir of dieting. It's essential for so many healthy reasons, the main one being the elimination of body wastes.

When I first started dieting, I began drinking a little water every day, mainly because it made my stomach feel full. Then, when I realized how good it tasted, I started drinking a few glasses every day.

For the last fifteen years, I've been drinking at least eight glasses of water a day, in addition to all the other fluids, such as coffee and juices, I drink.

Get yourself a big jug and start slurping.

Snacks

Every day between meals, when I'm hungry, I eat two or three pieces of fruit of whatever kind looks good, ripe, and juicy, in the store.

By now, you know I don't like vegetables very much. The only ones that taste any good to me are potatoes and corn, naturally. But I do eat carrots, celery, and tomatoes for the crunching and popping and for health reasons. I keep a supply cut up in my refrigerator.

Hot-air popcorn is my favorite. No butter, oil, or fats added. (Two quarts of this popcorn has less calories than 25 potato chips!)

Good luck and cheerful chewing.

DO'S

Get your doctor's approval for your weight goal and exercise program.

Ask your doctor about adding bran to your breakfast and about other high fiber foods you should eat each day.

Drink 6–8 glasses of water every day. (Other liquids are fine, but they don't count.)

Exercise 15 minutes, more if you have the time, each day.

Weigh yourself every day in the morning before eating.

Record your weight every day.

Eat a variety of foods on your diet.

Alternate chicken, turkey, fish. Enjoy lots of fresh fruits and vegetables.

Eat very, very s-l-o-w-l-y. Savor each bite.

Eat breakfast like a king, lunch like a prince, and dine like a pauper.

Be patient. Remember, this is a lifetime program, so give it time to work. You will lose weight, but you will have plateaus, too.

CONTROLLED CHEATING WORKS

DON'TS

Don't lie to yourself. Count every bit of food or drink that passes your lips.

Don't make excuses. If you goof, it's okay. Be honest, get back on the program immediately, and renew your commitment.

Except on your Cheating Day, do not eat pies, cakes, cookies, candies, fried foods, peanut butter, nuts, cheese, regular salad dressing, sugar, pickles, soups, dried fruit, or fast food.

Do not add salt to your food.

Do not eat very much red meat beef. Keep it to a minimum. Cut away all visible fat.

Do not eat unless you're hungry. A little hunger will help you lose weight.

Do not waste calories. Don't eat just to eat.

Do not change your Cheating Day.

Do not eat the skin on chicken or turkey.

Avoid fats and oils. Do not use more than one tablespoon each day.

CONTROLLED CHEATING WORKS

Goldberg's Short Cuts, Skinny Dips, Sweet Nothings, and Other Low-Calorie, Easy-Make Treats

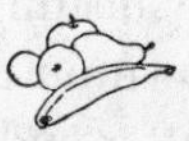

Here is a low-calorie recipe section of the book with yummy slim recipes for slimming people.

I'm an eater, not a cooker. Strolling into my kitchen, I took an inventory of all my cooking equipment. When I opened the oven door, two skinny angry moths were sitting on the dusty oven rack looking at me like an unwanted intruder. Nothing in there.

Underneath the oven, the sticky broiler door squeaked as if I was creeping into a haunted house. I'll be darned. There were twenty-seven foil pizza pans, two bent skillets for making fortune cookies, one half-melted plastic spatula, and one cheese-crusted oven rack for baking pizza cones.

Above the sink in my warped wood cabinets sat nineteen glasses, four knives, four forks, three teaspoons, four tablespoons, but no plates or bowls. I gave them to the Salvation Army four years ago. When I'm dining at home, I use elegant designer plastic-coated paper plates.

Next to the sink is my Rubbermaid dish drainer with one

Woolworth serrated-edge knife, one fork, one tablespoon, one teaspoon, and two glasses. All the eating tools came from Marshall Field's basement on a snowy Saturday afternoon in 1961.

This may sound weird coming from someone who likes to eat so much, but I don't like to cook. And reading cookbooks makes me hungry and bored. If I see one more recipe calling for ½ teaspoon of ginger, I'm going to pass out. I know that many former fatties love to horse around in the kitchen, but not me, baby. The only food I like to cook is pizza. It's such a simple fun food to make but the variations are endless. You can make whole-wheat, rye, bagel, or English-muffin dough, and try 689,043 different cheeses, toppings, and tomatoes.

Cheating Eating one night, when a full moon was beating down on my forehead and I was a little nutsy, I tried a peanut butter-and-jelly pizza. *Don't ask.* Whipping it out of the oven, it looked exactly as you might imagine melted peanut butter would look—and it tasted worse.

I had to do something. I needed some great recipes for all my Controlled Cheaters to use on those long lonely Diet Days. I had to call in the troops—the food and cooking experts who have the know-how to tease, please, and appease our appetites. I discovered that the federal government, various food associations, foundations, health groups, plus many food manufacturers, spend barrels of money creating low-calorie recipes. These recipes are developed by professional home economists and nutritionists and most are checked with consumer panels for taste and ease of making.

I spared no expense and called all over the country for the very best recipes. (You should see my phone bill.) I even wrote letters, which I hate to do, asking for the best recipes around. Finally, after getting about 500 recipes, I drafted such serious food folk as Bonnie Winston in Kansas City, Marlene Levinson in San Francisco, and Julie Davis in New York to pick out and kitchen-test the simple and most delicious recipes.

I dedicate this cookbook to all you Cooking Controlled Cheaters. Good luck. What time can I come over to your house to eat?

IN THE BEGINNING . . . BREAKFAST

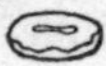

Banana Bonanza

1 medium banana
1 large egg
⅓ cup water
1½ tablespoons frozen orange juice concentrate
1 teaspoon wheat germ
1 teaspoon honey
Dash salt

Slice banana into blender jar. Add all remaining ingredients and blend at high speed for 1 minute.

Makes 1⅓ cups
Approximately 350 calories

Courtesy of Dole Bananas

Noisy Nut Cereal

3 cups rolled oats, quick-cooking
1 cup unsweetened wheat germ
½ cup coconut, flaked, or sunflower seeds, shelled
1 cup nuts, coarsely chopped
1 cup raisins
½ cup oil
½ cup honey
2 teaspoons vanilla

Preheat oven to 275° F. (very slow). Mix rolled oats, wheat germ, coconut or sunflower seeds, nuts, and raisins in a large bowl. Mix oil, honey, and vanilla. Pour over rolled oat mixture. Stir lightly until evenly mixed. Spread mixture on a 15-by-10-by-1-inch baking pan. Bake for 1 hour, stirring each 15 minutes. Cool. Break up any large lumps. Store in an airtight container.

Makes 15 servings, about ½ cup each
Calories per serving: about 280 with coconut;
290 with sunflower seeds

Courtesy of the U. S. Department of Agriculture

Saucy Shingle

¼ cup low-fat cottage cheese
½ cup unsweetened applesauce
1 slice bread
Pinch cinnamon or nutmeg

Mix cottage cheese and applesauce together. Spread on bread. Sprinkle with cinnamon or nutmeg. Toast in broiler or toaster-oven.

For one serving
163 calories

Strawberry Squirt

6 fresh ripe strawberries
1 cup vanilla yogurt
6½ ounces chilled club soda

Blend berries and yogurt at high speed until smooth. Stir in chilled club soda.

To make Strawberry Squirtsicle: Pour the Strawberry Squirt drink into a 4-ounce paper cup. Insert a wooden stick in the center and freeze. When frozen, peel off paper cup and eat as a frozen pop.

Approximately 250 calories

Courtesy Dannon Yogurt

THE LUNCH BUNCH

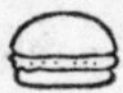

Tuna/Tomato Twosome

1 can (6½ ounces) chunk light tuna in water
½ cup chopped celery
⅓ cup imitation or low-calorie mayonnaise
¼ cup chopped parsley
2 tablespoons minced green onion
¼ teaspoon black pepper
36 cherry tomatoes
Parsley sprigs for garnish

Drain tuna. Combine tuna, celery, mayonnaise, chopped parsley, green onion, and pepper. Cut tops off tomatoes and scoop out seeds; turn upside down to drain. Fill with tuna salad. Serve chilled on parsley-lined plate.

Makes 36 portions
21 calories per portion

Courtesy of Bumble Bee Tuna

Manhattan Clam Chowder Cha Cha

3 cans (7 ounces each) minced clams
3 medium potatoes, peeled and diced
3 medium carrots, peeled and diced
4 medium stalks celery, chopped
1 can (16 ounces) tomatoes
1 tablespoon bacon-flavored bits
2 teaspoons salt
½ teaspoon thyme leaves
¼ teaspoon pepper

In a large kettle or Dutch oven, combine all ingredients and 4 cups water. Cover and simmer for 1 hour.

Makes 8 servings
About 100 calories each

Greater Tomato-Potato Salad

4 large tomatoes
1 medium potato, peeled, cooked, and diced
1 medium carrot, peeled and chopped
¼ cup low-fat cottage cheese
2 tablespoons chopped parsley
½ teaspoon salt

Cut tomatoes in half and scoop out centers to make cups. Strain pulp to remove excess liquid; reserve pulp. Pat insides of tomato cups with paper towels to dry. Combine reserved tomato pulp, potato, carrot, cottage cheese, parsley, and salt. Spoon mixture into tomato cups. Chill.

Makes 8 stuffed shells
About 40 calories each

TO DRESS A SLIM POTATO SALAD

Tomato juice with a hint of herbs or
Vinaigrette dressing: vinegar and just a dash of oil or
Mustard and a dab of sour cream or
Herb-dressed yogurt or
A splash of dry white wine

Courtesy of The Potato Board

Cheese and Noodle Doodle

1 package (8 ounces) broad noodles
3 tablespoons margarine
1½ cups low-fat cottage cheese
1 cup plain low-fat yogurt
4 teaspoons flour
1 teaspoon salt
Dash pepper
½ cup light raisins
4 egg whites, stiffly beaten
3 tablespoons fine dry bread crumbs

Cook noodles in salted water for 8 minutes; drain and turn into a large bowl. Add margarine and mix well. Mix cottage cheese, yogurt, flour, salt, pepper, and raisins in small bowl; add to noodles and mix well. Fold in beaten egg whites. Turn into shallow 2-quart baking dish that has been brushed with margarine. Sprinkle bread crumbs evenly over top. Bake in 375° F. oven for 30 minutes, or until lightly browned. Serve with additional yogurt.

Makes 8 servings
Approximately 200 calories a serving

Courtesy of Promise Margarine

*Mary Had a Little Salad**

3 cups cold cooked rice
2 cups cubed cooked lamb
1 medium tomato, diced
½ cup each: chopped red onion and chopped parsley
½ cup bottled low-calorie Italian salad dressing
3 tablespoons lemon juice
Salt
Pepper
Salad greens

Combine all ingredients except salad greens in bowl. Mix well and chill. Serve on salad greens.

Makes 6 servings
Approximately 277 calories a serving

Courtesy Lamb Education Center

* Mary had a little salad
It had lamb and rice
Every time she made it,
She said, "This is so nice!"

Toutes-Les-Fruits Salad

1 Golden Delicious apple,
cored and sliced
1 Red Delicious apple,
cored and sliced
1 fresh pineapple,
peeled and cut into spears
1 small honeydew melon,
peeled and cut into chunks
1 orange, peeled and sliced
Salad greens
Lemon slices
Lemon Yogurt Dressing*

Prepare fruits and arrange on large lettuce-lined platter. Garnish with lemon slices. Serve with Lemon Yogurt Dressing.

Makes 8 servings
Approximately 130 calories a serving

*LEMON YOGURT DRESSING

1 cup plain yogurt
1 tablespoon lemon juice
½ teaspoon grated lemon rind
¼ teaspoon non-nutritive sweetener

Combine all ingredients; mix well.

Makes 1 cup

Courtesy Washington Apples

Garden of Eatin' Salad

1½ cups cooked sliced carrots
1½ cups cooked whole or cut green beans
1½ cups cooked green peas
1 cup sliced celery
1 small onion, chopped
½ cup Spanish stuffed green olives
⅓ cup plain yogurt
2 tablespoons chili sauce
½ teaspoon lemon juice
¼ teaspoon salt
Boston lettuce

Chill vegetables and olives in large bowl. Combine yogurt, chili sauce, lemon juice, and salt. Just before serving, toss yogurt dressing with vegetables. Line serving bowl with lettuce leaves and spoon salad into center.

Makes 6 servings
83 calories each

Courtesy Spanish Green Olive Commission

California Walking Salad

1 pound seedless grapes, pulled from stems
1 red apple, cored and cubed
½ cup raisins
¼ cup toasted slivered almonds
1 head iceberg lettuce, cored, rinsed, drained, and chilled

In a bowl, mix grapes, apple, raisins, and almonds. Carefully remove lettuce leaves from head, one at a time. Put ½ cup of the fruit-nut mixture in each lettuce cup. Serve out of hand.

Makes 6 to 8 salads
Approximately 130 calories a serving

Courtesy California Table Grape Commission

Veggie-Scallop Salad

1½ pounds scallops, fresh or frozen
1 quart boiling water
2 tablespoons salt
1 can (1 pound) cut green beans, drained
1 cup sliced celery
¼ cup chopped onion
¼ cup chopped green pepper
1 tablespoon chopped pimiento
Marinade*
6 lettuce cups

Thaw frozen scallops. Rinse with cold water to remove any shell particles. Place in boiling salted water. Cover and return to the boiling point. Reduce heat and simmer for 3 to 4 minutes, depending on size. Drain and cool. Slice scallops. Combine all ingredients except lettuce. Cover and chill for at least 1 hour. Drain. Serve in lettuce cups.

Makes 6 servings
Approximately 140 calories a serving

*MARINADE

½ cup cider vinegar
1 tablespoon sugar
¼ teaspoon salt
Dash pepper
¼ cup salad oil

Combine vinegar, sugar, salt, and pepper. Add oil gradually, blending thoroughly.

Makes approximately ⅔ cup marinade

Courtesy of the National Marine Fisheries Service

Sandwich Spectaculars

Beef 'n' Cheese

½ cup plain yogurt
¼ cup crumbled Blue cheese
8 thin slices cooked roast beef
Softened butter
8 slices pumpernickel bread
Lettuce
8 cherry tomatoes, cut in half
8 cucumber slices

In a bowl combine the yogurt and Blue cheese. Spread about 1 tablespoon on each slice roast beef. Roll jelly-roll fashion. Butter bread. Arrange lettuce, then a beef roll on each slice. Top with 2 cherry tomato halves. Cut cucumber slices in half; twist and serve as a garnish.

Makes 8 sandwiches
201 calories a sandwich

Shrimp 'n' Egg

4 hard-cooked eggs
¼ cup dairy sour cream
¼ teaspoon celery salt
¼ cup (½ stick) butter
1 teaspoon curry powder
3 tablespoons coarsely chopped watercress
8 thin slices square pumpernickel bread
Pimiento, cut in designs
16 large cooked shrimp, cut in half lengthwise
Capers

Slice eggs crosswise; set aside 8 center slices. Finely chop the remaining egg and fold into the sour cream along with the celery salt; set aside. In a small mixing bowl beat the butter and curry powder together until fluffy; fold in the watercress. Spread the butter on one side of each slice of bread, then spread on about 3 tablespoons of the egg mixture. Place a slice of reserved egg in the center and top with pimiento. Arrange 1 shrimp half in each corner and garnish with capers. Refrigerate until served.

Makes 8 sandwiches
209 calories a sandwich

Courtesy United Dairy Industry Association

LEAN IN-BETWEENS

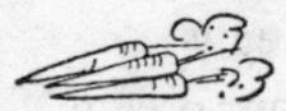

Mean Joe's Greens

⅓ cup salad oil
⅓ cup cider vinegar
2 tablespoons green pepper, finely chopped
1 tablespoon parsley, chopped
1 teaspoon salt
¼ teaspoon paprika
⅛ teaspoon pepper
3 cups (1 small head) cauliflower, broken into florets, cooked tender-crisp
15-ounce can garbanzo beans, heated, drained
2 cups cucumber, unpared, sliced
1 cup carrots, cut in thin strips

Place oil, vinegar, green pepper, parsley, salt, and spices in a large bowl. Mix well. Add vegetables and mix gently. Cover. Marinate for several hours or overnight in the refrigerator. Stir occasionally. For optimum eating quality, use within a few days.

Makes 7 cups
About 75 calories per ½ cup

Courtesy of the U. S. Department of Agriculture

Make-a-Rumaki

6 chicken livers, washed, dried, halved
1 tablespoon horseradish mustard
4 bacon slices, cut in thirds
6 water chestnuts, cut in halves

Mix livers with horseradish mustard. Wrap each bacon strip around a piece of liver and a water chestnut half. Secure with a toothpick. Broil, turning frequently, until bacon is crisp, about 10 to 15 minutes.

NOTE: Use round wooden toothpicks for this recipe. Flat toothpicks may char during broiling.

Makes 12 rumaki
Calories per rumaki: about 30

Courtesy of the U. S. Department of Agriculture

Ricotta Picasso Swirls

1 cup ricotta
1 clove garlic, finely minced
2 tablespoons freshly minced parsley
1 teaspoon salt
1 teaspoon basil
1 teaspoon freshly grated lemon peel
½ teaspoon thyme
Celery sticks
Cucumber rounds

In a small bowl, combine the ricotta, garlic, parsley, salt, basil, lemon peel, and thyme. Mix well. Refrigerate for at least 1 hour to allow flavors to blend. Assemble and fill electric foodgun according to manufacturer's instructions; fit with decorator tip; use Lo Speed. With fork or fingers to steady vegetables, pipe a swirl of filling onto each piece of celery or cucumber. Garnish as desired.

Makes 1 cup of filling
Approximately 500 calories

Courtesy Wear-Ever Aluminum

Apple Shrimp Kabobs

2 Golden Delicious apples
2 dozen medium shrimp, cooked, peeled, and deveined
½ cup bottled low-calorie Italian dressing
¼ cup lemon juice
Parsley

Core apples and cut each into 8 wedges. Cut each wedge into 3 bite-size pieces. Toss apples and shrimp with dressing and lemon juice. Marinate about 1 hour. Drain, reserving marinade for another use. Arrange 2 apple chunks and 1 shrimp on small skewers or cocktail picks. Place on serving plate and garnish with parsley.

Makes 24 appetizers
Approximately 30 calories an appetizer

Courtesy Washington Apples

Ambrosia Apple Dip

1 cup cottage cheese
¼ teaspoon non-nutritive sweetener
1 teaspoon grated orange peel
3 tablespoons orange juice
¼ teaspoon ginger
2 tablespoons coconut
Red and Golden Delicious apple wedges

Blend cottage cheese in blender until smooth. Add sugar substitute, orange peel, juice, and ginger. Blend until well mixed. Stir in coconut. Chill. Serve as dip for apple wedges.

Makes 1¼ cups dip
Approximately 500 calories

Courtesy Washington Apples

My Blue Heaven Cheese Dressing

1 cup plain yogurt
⅓ cup (1¼ ounces) crumbled Blue cheese
Grated peel and juice of ½ fresh lemon
1 small clove garlic, minced
½ teaspoon seasoned salt
⅛ teaspoon pepper

Combine all ingredients and chill. Serve over crisp salad greens.

Makes about 1 cup
(16 calories a tablespoon)

VARIATION: Serve as a dip with assorted raw vegetables.

Courtesy Sunkist Growers Inc.

Popcorn

I bought one of those hot-air popcorn poppers when I found out that popcorn, when it's not popped in oils and is left unbuttered after those little kernels are popped, has only 25 to 55 calories per cup, depending on the size of the popped kernel. Another reason was that the hot-air popper was on sale for $16. I figured that if I started eating too much popcorn, I could always use it as a hair dryer or hand warmer or refrigerator defroster.

Good old popcorn is a whole grain, super-nutritious and a good source of fiber.

If you don't want to spring for a hot-air popcorn popper, you can use any old skillet or pan with a lid. For a little exercise, leave the lid off and run around the kitchen, trying to catch the popped corn in your mouth as it flies out of the pan.

Someone told me yesterday that you can pop corn in your microwave oven. And that they even have special poppers to do it. Land O'Goldberg, what won't they think of next?

DINNER WINNERS

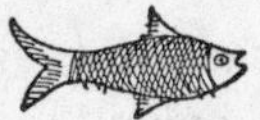

Wok Around the Clock Lamb

1 tablespoon diet margarine
1 pound lean leg or shoulder lamb, trimmed of fat and cut into thin strips
1 onion, thinly sliced
1 clove garlic, minced
1 green pepper, cut into 1½-inch strips
1 cup diagonally cut celery slices
1 cup very thinly sliced carrots
1 cup fresh, sliced mushrooms
1 cup fresh bean sprouts
1 package (6 ounces) frozen snow pea pods
2 tablespoons soy sauce
2 teaspoons cornstarch
½ cup chicken or beef bouillon
⅛ teaspoon pepper
1 teaspoon sugar

Melt margarine in non-stick skillet or wok. Add lamb and brown quickly. Add onion, garlic, green pepper, celery, and carrots. Cook, stirring constantly, until vegetables are crisp-tender. Add mushrooms, bean sprouts, and snow pea pods. Mix together soy sauce, cornstarch, bouillon, pepper, and sugar. Pour over lamb and vegetables. Cook, stirring constantly, for just a few minutes.

Makes 4 servings
Approximately 260 calories a serving

Courtesy of The American Lamb Council

Orange You Glad We Thought of This Recipe?

2 tablespoons margarine
½ cup chopped onion
2 large tomatoes, peeled, seeded, and chopped
½ cup orange juice
1 teaspoon salt
½ teaspoon dried leaf savory or thyme
1 pound flounder fillets, fresh or frozen

In a medium saucepan melt margarine. Add onion and cook until tender. Add tomatoes and simmer for 10 minutes. Add orange juice, salt, and savory. Simmer 5 minutes. Set aside.

Roll flounder fillets and place in a shallow baking dish, seam side down. Pour orange-tomato sauce over rolls. Bake in 350° F. oven for 25 minutes, or until fish flakes easily when tested with a fork.

Makes 4 servings
Approximately 200 calories a serving

Courtesy of Promise Margarine

On the Lamb

1 or 2 green peppers, cut into 1- to 1½-inch squares
4 stalks celery, cut into 1- to 1½-inch squares
3 large carrots, cut into 1-inch pieces
½ pound fresh mushrooms
1½ pounds lean lamb, cut into ¾-inch cubes
1½ teaspoons salt
Dash black pepper
3 cups tomato sauce
¾ teaspoon whole cloves
Dash oregano
2 tablespoons Worcestershire sauce

Parboil green peppers, celery, carrots, and mushrooms for 10 minutes. Arrange meat and vegetables on skewers. Place skewers of meat and vegetables in a single layer in roasting pans. Sprinkle with salt and pepper. Combine tomato sauce, cloves, oregano, and Worcestershire sauce; pour over kebabs. Bake at 325° F. for 30 to 45 minutes, or until done. Baste frequently with pan liquid.

Makes 6 servings
Each serving is approximately 275 calories

Courtesy Lamb Education Center

Turkey Orient Express

2 tablespoons margarine
2 tablespoons oil
1 teaspoon paprika
6 turkey wings
¾ teaspoon salt
¼ teaspoon pepper
4 tablespoons sesame seeds, divided

Melt margarine in 9- x 13-inch baking dish; stir in oil and paprika. Add turkey wings, turning once. Sprinkle with salt, pepper, and half of sesame seeds. Bake at 350° F. for 30 minutes. Turn wings again and sprinkle with remaining seeds. Bake for 30 minutes, or until tender. Serve with Mandarin Sauce.

Makes 6 servings
Calories: 108 per serving

MANDARIN SAUCE

1 cup orange juice
½ cup currant or apple jelly
1 teaspoon lemon juice
¼ teaspoon ginger
1 tablespoon cornstarch
1 can (11 ounces) mandarin oranges, drained

Combine first five ingredients in small saucepan. Heat and stir until smooth and clear. Remove from heat. Stir in mandarin oranges.

Makes 6 servings
Calories: 108 per serving

Courtesy Turkey Information Service

A Wing and a Pear

1 can (16 ounces) Bartlett pear halves
1 (2- to 2½-pound) broiler-fryer, cut up, remove skin
Salt and pepper
1 medium onion, sliced
1 tablespoon oil
3 tablespoons flour
½ teaspoon basil
¾ cup water
⅓ cup dry white wine
1 cup halved cherry tomatoes

Drain and quarter pears, reserving ⅓ cup pear syrup. Sprinkle chicken pieces with salt and pepper. Brown chicken under broiler. Remove to casserole. Saute sliced onion until tender in oil in skillet. Blend in flour and basil. Add water gradually, cooking and stirring until thickened and bubbly. Add reserved pear syrup and white wine. Add pears and tomatoes and cook for a few minutes longer. Season to taste with salt and pepper. Pour pear sauce over chicken in casserole. Cover and bake at 350° F. for 45 minutes, or until chicken is tender, removing cover for last 5 minutes.

Makes 4 servings
Approximately 375 calories per serving

Courtesy Pacific Coast Canned Pear Service

Chili Chicken Quickie (Tostada de Pollo)

2 cans (7 ounces each) green chili salsa
1 medium onion, chopped
1 medium clove garlic, minced
Grated peel and juice of ½ fresh lemon
1½ cups cooked chicken cut in small pieces
4 (8-inch) flour tortillas
1 cup (about 4 ounces) shredded cheese
Shredded lettuce
2 small tomatoes, sliced or cubed
Taco sauce (optional)

In large skillet, combine salsa, onion, garlic, lemon peel and juice; simmer for 20 minutes, or until onion is tender. Add chicken and heat. Meanwhile, crisp tortillas by lightly browning each tortilla on both sides in a griddle, non-stick skillet, or broiler; keep warm. Place tortillas on plates; spoon chicken mixture on tortillas. Top with cheese, lettuce, and tomatoes. Serve with taco sauce.

Makes 4 servings
371 calories per serving

Courtesy Sunkist Growers Inc.

Unstout Trout

4 whole dressed, fresh or frozen Idaho Rainbow Trout
1 (8-ounce) bottle clam juice, or 1 cup chicken broth
2 tablespoons minced onions
1 tablespoon cooking oil
1 teaspoon Worcestershire sauce
¼ teaspoon salt
⅛ teaspoon oregano
⅛ teaspoon thyme
⅛ teaspoon pepper
3 cups steamed julienned vegetables; any of these combinations—carrots, green beans, celery, turnips, or zucchini
Lemon and chopped parsley

Thaw trout if frozen. Bone trout if necessary: Position the trout on a platter in front of you with the head facing left if you're right-handed. Slip a butter knife along the entire length of the backbone, steadying the fish with a fork in your left hand. Gently lift away the top fillet, including bones and tail. Use the knife to separate the head from the bottom fillet; flip the top fillet over, skin side down, on the platter. Lift away bone structure. In a saucepan, combine clam juice, onion, oil, Worcestershire sauce, and seasonings. Boil liquid rapidly for approximately 5 minutes, reducing it to ½ cup. Place opened fish skin side down on a well-oiled broiler rack. Brush trout with sauce. Broil 3 inches from heat for about 5 minutes. Brush trout with sauce once or twice while broiling. Carefully lift trout from broiler and center on a warm platter. Surround with vegetables. Serve with lemon and sprinkle with chopped parsley, if desired.

Makes 4 servings
Approximately 340 calories per serving

United States Trout Farmers Association

Chew Man Chinese Pepper Steak

1¼ pounds top round steak, cut ¾ to 1 inch thick*
1 tablespoon cornstarch
½ teaspoon sugar
¼ teaspoon ginger
¼ cup soy sauce
3 medium green peppers
3 small tomatoes
2 tablespoons cooking oil
1 clove garlic, minced
¼ cup water

Partially freeze steak to firm and slice diagonally across the grain into very thin strips. Combine cornstarch, sugar, and ginger and stir in soy sauce. Pour mixture over meat and stir. Cut green peppers into thin strips and cut tomatoes into wedges. Quickly brown beef strips (⅓ at a time) in hot oil and remove from pan. Reduce heat; add green pepper, garlic, and water to pan and cook until green pepper is tender-crisp, 5 to 6 minutes. Stir in meat and tomatoes and heat through.

Makes 4 servings
Approximately 400 calories per serving

Courtesy National Live Stock & Meat Board

* 1 flank steak (approximately 1¼ pounds) can be used.

DON'T DESERT DESSERT

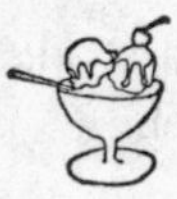

Yes We Have Some Banana Frozen Yogurt

3 bananas
1 tablespoon lemon juice
1 envelope unflavored gelatin
½ cup sugar
⅛ teaspoon salt
3 containers (8 ounces each) plain yogurt

In a 5-cup blender container, purée bananas with lemon juice. In medium saucepan mix unflavored gelatin with sugar and salt. Blend 1 cup banana purée into gelatin mixture; let stand 1 minute. Stir over low heat until gelatin is completely dissolved, about 5 minutes. Remove from heat; cool slightly. Stir in yogurt. Turn into freezer can of 2- or 4-quart ice cream maker. Insert dasher; cover, freeze according to manufacturer's directions. Pour into 2-quart container; allow to ripen about 2 hours in freezer.

FREEZER TRAY METHOD

Pour banana-yogurt mixture into freezer tray or 9- x 5- x 3-inch loaf pan. Freeze until firm. Turn frozen mixture into large bowl, add 2 unbeaten egg whites. Beat at high speed in electric mixer until smooth and fluffy, about 10 minutes. Return to pan and freeze.

Makes about 2 quarts
Approximately 1,600 calories for 2 quarts

Courtesy of The Banana Bunch

Lean Lemon Cheesecake

CRUST

½ cup corn flakes
1 tablespoon melted margarine
1 tablespoon granulated sugar
Dash of salt

FILLING

12 ounces creamed cottage cheese
2 eggs
½ cup granulated sugar
½ teaspoon lemon extract

Preheat oven to 350° F. Mix all the crust ingredients together and spread on the bottom and up the sides of an 8-inch pie plate. Pour all filling ingredients into a blender and blend until smooth. Pour mixture into the pie shell. Bake for 35 minutes, or until filling puffs and seems dry on top. Cool for 15 minutes. Refrigerate for 2 hours. Garnish with lemon and orange rind.

Makes 8 servings
Approximately 900 calories for the whole cheesecake

Courtesy of the American Diabetes Association

Custard's Last Stand

1 can (16 ounces) water-packed pear halves
1 can (11 ounces) water-packed mandarin orange segments
¼ cup lemon juice
¼ teaspoon salt
Artificial sweetener to equal 3 tablespoons sugar
2 tablespoons cornstarch
1 egg, well-beaten
½ teaspoon grated lemon peel

Drain fruits, reserving juice. Cut pears in half, lengthwise. Measure syrups to make 1½ cups. Combine fruit juice, lemon juice, salt, sweetener, and cornstarch in small saucepan. Cook, stirring constantly, until thickened and bubbly. Add small amount of hot mixture to well-beaten egg and blend thoroughly. Return to hot mixture and cook, stirring, 1 minute longer. Remove from heat and add grated lemon peel. Cool. Place small amount of lemon custard in bottom of four sherbet glasses. Arrange pears, spoke-fashion, in custard. Place orange segments in center, reserving a few for garnish. Divide remaining custard over fruit. Garnish with reserved orange segments. Chill.

Makes 4 servings
Approximately 120 calories per serving

Courtesy Pacific Coast Canned Pear Service

Cool Coffee Soufflé

1 envelope unflavored gelatin (1 tablespoon)
1 tablespoon instant coffee
⅓ cup sugar
¼ to ½ teaspoon cinnamon
1 cup boiling water
6 eggs, separated

Make a 4-inch band of triple-thickness wax paper long enough to go around a soufflé dish and overlap 2 inches. Wrap around outside of dish. Fasten with tape, string, or paper clip. (Collar should extend 2 inches above rim of dish.) Set aside. In medium bowl stir together gelatin, coffee, sugar, and cinnamon. Add boiling water and stir until coffee and sugar dissolve. Cool slightly. Beat yolks until light and lemon-colored; stir into gelatin mixture. Chill, stirring occasionally, until mixture mounds slightly when dropped from spoon, 30 to 45 minutes. Wash beaters. In large mixing bowl beat egg whites until stiff but not dry, just until whites no longer slip when bowl is tilted. Gently but thoroughly fold chilled gelatin mixture into egg whites. Carefully pour into prepared dish. Chill until firm, 3 to 4 hours. Just before serving, carefully remove wax paper collar.

Makes 6 servings
Approximately 750 calories for the soufflé

Courtesy American Egg Board

Lighten Up Lemon Soufflé

6 eggs, separated
⅔ cup water
⅓ cup lemon juice
Dash salt
1 envelope unflavored gelatin
1 tablespoon grated lemon peel
½ teaspoon cream of tartar
⅓ cup sugar

Make 4-inch band of triple-thickness aluminum foil long enough to go around a 1- or 1½-quart* soufflé dish and overlap 2

* An aluminum band is not required on 1½-quart dish.

inches. Wrap around outside of dish. Fasten with tape, paper clip, or string. Collar should extend 2 inches above rim of dish. Set aside. In medium saucepan, beat egg yolks with water, lemon juice, and salt. Sprinkle gelatin over yolk mixture and let stand 1 minute. Stir over low heat until gelatin is completely dissolved, about 5 to 7 minutes. Remove from heat. Stir in lemon peel. Chill, stirring occasionally, until mixture mounds slightly when dropped from spoon, 30 to 45 minutes. In large bowl, beat egg whites with cream of tartar at high speed until foamy. Beat in sugar, 1 tablespoon at a time, until sugar is dissolved** and whites are glossy and stand in soft peaks. Gently but thoroughly fold in chilled gelatin mixture. Pile into prepared dish. Chill until firm, several hours or overnight. To serve, remove aluminum band. Variation: Spoon soufflé mixture into 6 individual dessert dishes and chill.

Makes 6 servings
Approximately 140 calories per serving

Courtesy American Egg Board

Out! Out! Damn Calories! Piña Custards

4 eggs, slightly beaten
3 tablespoons granulated brown sugar artificially flavored replacement
1½ teaspoons vanilla
Artificial sweetener to equal ⅓ cup sugar
¼ teaspoon salt
3 cups skim milk or reconstituted instant non-fat dry milk, heated until very warm
6 slices pineapple, packed in own juice, drained
Nutmeg, optional

** Rub just a bit of meringue between thumb and forefinger to feel if sugar has dissolved.

Mix together eggs, brown sugar replacement, vanilla, sweetener, and salt. Gradually stir in milk. Pour into six (6-ounce) custard cups. Top with pineapple slices.* Sprinkle with nutmeg, if desired. Set in 9- x 13- x 2-inch, or other large, baking pan. Pour very hot water into the pan to within ½ inch of the top of the custard. Bake in a preheated 350° F. oven until a knife inserted near the center comes out clean, 30 to 35 minutes. Remove promptly from hot water. Serve warm or chilled.

Makes 6 servings, about 140 calories each
Approximately 825 calories for the whole custard

Courtesy American Egg Board

Blintz Blitz

6 ounces cottage cheese
⅙ teaspoon artificial sweetener
A little cinnamon
Capful of vanilla
4 slices extra thin sliced bread with crusts removed
2 eggs, beaten

Mix cottage cheese with artificial sweetener, cinnamon, and vanilla. Roll bread with a rolling pin and fill with one-quarter of the filling. Roll like a jelly roll. Dip each roll in egg, "fry" in a Teflon pan.

Approximately 110 calories per blintz

* Pineapple slices may be placed on custard after baking, if desired.

Brownie Blast

2 cups fine graham cracker crumbs (about 24 crackers)
½ cup chopped walnuts
3 ounces semisweet chocolate pieces
1½ teaspoons artificial sweetener
¼ teaspoon salt
1 cup skim milk

Preheat oven to 350° F. Place all ingredients in bowl and stir until blended. Turn into a greased 8- x 8- x 2-inch pan. Bake for 30 minutes. Cut into 2-inch squares while warm.

Makes 16

1 brownie equals 95 calories

Courtesy of Cumberland Packing Corp.,
Manufacturers of Sweet 'N Low Brand
Granulated Sugar Substitute

Carmen Miran-Dish

1 grapefruit
1 orange
1 apple
2 cups diced honeydew or cantaloupe (about ½ melon)
¼ cup red maraschino cherries, drained
Confectioners' sugar
2 tablespoons shredded coconut

Peel grapefruit and orange, holding over bowl to catch juice; cut fruit into sections. Core unpeeled apple; cut into bite-size pieces. Combine fruit in bowl with juice and toss. If desired, sweeten to taste with about 1 tablespoon confectioners' sugar. Cover and chill until ready to serve, at least 1 hour.

Just before serving, spoon into 6 serving dishes and sprinkle about 1 teaspoon coconut over each. Garnish with additional stemmed cherries, if desired.

Makes 6 servings
About 140 calories each

Courtesy Cherry Growers and Industries Foundation

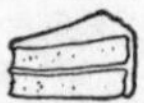

Cheatin' Eatin'

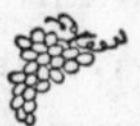

Congrats, wowee, zap, zoweee, you've made it to your first Controlled Cheating Day. In all your natural (no additives), long healthy life, you will never have to diet for longer than six days without cheating.

Turn around real quick and look back on the last fourteen days. You can do this a lot easier now because you've even lost pounds and inches off your shoulders. Those days weren't too tough for a low-cal cookie like you, were they? Your diet gave you plenty to eat. It was balanced and all those nourishing nutrients energized you enough to roof the house with one-inch squares, mow the lawn with a pair of scissors, and play three sets of tennis with a racquet with no strings, all on Saturday morning before eleven-thirty.

That diet, plus all those nifty food substitutions you can move around and up and down the diet, will slay that old diet dragon, boredom, with the Golden Sword of Variety. Even when your Controlled Cheating Day is over, you can return to your diet without a whimper or a tear.

CONTROLLED CHEATING IS HEALTHY

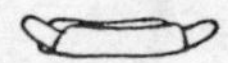

The biggest, largest, grandest reason I know Controlled Cheating is healthy is that I'm sitting here on a rainy Saturday afternoon staring at my humming Smith-Corona and pounding away with my ten bony fingers.

When I was fat, the doctors said I'd be lucky to reach thirty. I'm now forty-seven years old, in the best shape of my life, except for an occasional stretch mark, and I never get sick. Once in a while I do get a sore throat—but that's from keeping my head too long in ice cream freezers.

When I was growing up and also spreading out (I weighed 105 pounds in the third grade and 240 in the eighth grade), I went to a couple of doctors. My very own pediatrician hauled me up on the examining table one day. (I had to help because he was afraid of straining himself.) He asked if I wanted to die from overeating in ten years. Not having been formally introduced to death at the age of ten, I became a screaming hypochondriac.

The hypochondria got so bad by the time I was in college that a friend had to rip the Medicine section out of *Time* magazine before I could read it. As soon as I started losing weight, I lost the hypochondria, too. Now I'm thin and cured.

But back to the doctors. They all said the same thing: "Goldberg, you sure do like your groceries. You've got to lose weight. Instead of a Tootsie Roll, pick up an apple." They didn't know who they were talking to. I thought the only apples in the world were grown in Dutch apple pie with a sugary, crunchy top with raisins and heavy cinnamon.

Then these same M.D.s would hand me the usual mimeographed sheet with the usual diet. The diet was always the same. Breakfast: half a grapefruit, one soft-boiled egg, one piece of dry whole-wheat toast, a glass of skim milk, and coffee or tea with no sugar or cream. Lunch and dinner were even more terrible. I was supposed to stay on THAT the rest of my life?

But I always started the following morning with mighty resolve. By 8:35 A.M. I had both hands rammed in a sack of nutty danishes. That blew that diet for another seven months.

Almost every medical, nutritional, and diet expert I've talked to, read about, and seen or heard gives the same advice to folks who want to lose weight and keep it off: Don't eliminate any food from your diet; rather, cut down the quantities you eat. That's wise advice, IF you can control yourself twenty-four hours a day, seven days a week, twelve months of every year of your life. I can't.

What they don't understand is how true fat people eat. There's not a chubby alive who can stop eating a hunk of fresh banana cake with chocolate ice cream after four bites. If they put a tiny sliver on the plate with a thimble of ice cream, it *will not* satisfy a real fatty. If a plumperoo could eat that way, he wouldn't be fat in the first place.

No one ever sat down and figured out how fat people eat. I had to think it through because I was going nowhere with every other diet plan. If I didn't, I knew in my soul that I would keep blowing up until I was the size of the Goodyear Blimp and explode in a couple of years.

I did take their health advice, but I switched it all around. I kept all the good stuff confined to one day a week for starters. Then I could be a free man in the morning when the diet began.

Bang. Controlled Cheating leaped in on little pig's feet. I saved all my Controlled Cheating calories for one outstanding day a week and ate everything and anything my heart desired.

At that moment, my 325-pound body wobbled with joy at the coming good health and sighed deeply with relief at the prospect of the 175-pound licorice anvil I was going to lift off its back. Everyone was happy.

CONTROLLED CHEATING FLIPS YOUR LID OR TAKES OFF YOUR DIETER'S DERBY

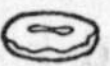

You're wearing an invisible, tight-fitting hat. You don't see it but, boy, you *can* feel it. I call it the Dieter's Derby, and it's automatically crammed on anyone who ever thought about pouring a fist full of cashews into their mouth. The Dieter's Derby comes only in black—with no feather. There are no pinks, chartreuses, or mauves. The Derby is not something you wear to the Easter Parade.

The mind-numbing tightness comes from always having to think about what you're going to eat and how many calories it has. Will the needle shoot up when you jump on the scale tomorrow morning? Do you really want that hot dog with sauerkraut? Sam or Samantha said you were getting a little heavy, shoot, are you going to eat that bag of chocolate chip cookies or not? Decisions, decisions, decisions.

See, there's this constant tension from always having to think about dieting and losing weight, and making decisions on what and how much you're going to eat. That ugly-as-mud Dieter's Derby was one of my biggest problems. All the other diets I'd been on were for seven horrible days and nights a week of endless weeks. My head was like a giant volcano ready to explode with strawberry milk shake pouring down my slopes. No relief was in sight.

Finally I discovered Controlled Cheating and the Dieter's Derby disappeared. Yes, just like at the West Point and Annapolis graduating ceremonies, you can throw your Dieter's Derby in the air and it evaporates on your Controlled Cheating Days. With Controlled Cheating Days all the tautness, pressure, and tightness are gone.

As Humphrey Yogurt once said, "Hat's off to you, kid."

CONTROLLED CHEATING IS GUILT-FREE

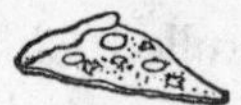

The Skinny World vs. Tammy and Teddy Thunder Thighs

JUDGE CRACKER: "Jury, have you reached a verdict?"

JURY: "Yes, your Honor, we have. We find the defendants guilty on all charges.

1. Eating a Wonder bread and Miracle Whip salami sandwich and washing it down with a lemon ice cream Kool Aid while supposedly on a diet.
2. Sneaking three tablespoons of turkey dressing at 2:30 A.M. on Thanksgiving morning, 1965.
3. Lifting four and a half French fries from their daughter Tara's plate at McDonald's.
4. Scraping the top off of three slices of sausage and pepperoni pizza while screaming, 'I never eat the crust; it's so fattening.' Then four minutes later starting to nibble until all three crusts were gone."

JUDGE CRACKER: "The jury has found you guilty on all counts. Do you have anything to say in your defense before I pass sentence?"

T & T: "Yes, your Honor. Who squealed?"

JUDGE CRACKER: "That's it? I should sentence both of you to a life term of gooey guilt, to be served in the Fat Slammer of Dumb Diets. However, being merciful, I will parole both of you to Controlled Cheating. Your parole officer to be General Goldberg."

T & T: "Oh, thank you, thank you. We look forward to it. Huzzah, huzzah for Judge Cracker."

Controlled Cheating *will* take all the guilt from Cheating Eating because it is *planned.* You know what you're going to do seven days a week. Controlled Cheating takes the tremendous weight of gooey guilt off your mind and stomach. Even without losing a pound the first day of your diet, you'll feel tons lighter.

For the first twenty-five years of my life, I carried around enough guilt about eating to make the gang in Sing Sing look as innocent as the Osmonds. Snatching handfuls of Hydrox Cookies from Goldberg's Market, running to the back room and stuffing them down: guilty. Stealing money from my thrifty, skinny sister Jocelyn to buy chocolate ice cream sodas with vanilla ice cream: guilty. Grabbing meatloaf from friends' plates in high school when they left to get a glass of water: guilty. Riffling the drawers of fraternity brothers at 2:00 A.M., when they got a goody package from home: guilty. Making homesick campers cry at Boy Scout Camp in Osceola, Missouri, so they couldn't eat and I could clean their plates: guilty.

But don't put the cuffs on me yet–I've repented. I used to feel guilty, but no more. Why? Because guilt from eating comes from uncontrollable eating when you aren't supposed to. With Controlled Cheating, you know what you're doing every minute of every day, especially on your Cheating Day when you've planned the one big day you're going to cheat and all of the goodies you're going to eat.

What a relief!

YOU AIN'T SUPPOSED TO MESS WITH YOUR CONTROLLED CHEATIN' DAY, NO HOW

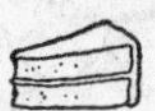

Once you've made the rock-hard choice of what Cheating Day you want, *that day cannot change.* Not for now, anyway. I want you to wait until you're firmly in the Controlled Cheating groove before we talk about that. Let me give you the reasons.

Suppose you've picked Saturday for your Controlled Cheating Day. Every Saturday you wake up happy as a hot dog in yellow mustard. Your Controlled Cheating Program is doing fine. You're losing weight and feeling great. Then comes an invitation for a Sunday outdoor barbecue of sirloin steaks, homemade potato salad, baked beans with brown sugar, fresh baked bread, tart cherry pie, and three barrels of cold beer.

STOP! Wait a minute. You *cannot* change your Cheating Eating Day.

I know you because I'm just like you. When you start switching Controlled Cheating Days for every dog fight and worm wrestle, you're headed for big Trouble with a capital T.

You'll not only cheat on that special Cheating Day, you'll cheat again on your regular Cheating Eating Day.

Right now you're in a happy groove. Don't mess around with success. Otherwise you'll be back ramming it in every day with both fists like you did before. Us fatties are sneaky.

The reason why Controlled Cheating works 100 percent of the time is that you can get through the toughest, hungriest days of your life because you can look forward to that wonderful Cheating Eating Day. It's special. Keep it that way. Savor it and you will not feel deprived, self-pitying, hurt, or martyred because you've got that one hot fudge sundae day on the horizon.

I know it's a rigid life now, but it's a happy, thin life and eventually you'll have more flexibility—I promise.

FATS GOLDBERG'S HIT LIST

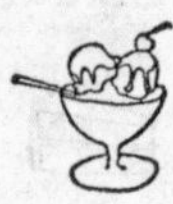

Your Cheating Day is here. All the preliminary matches are over and it's time to rip the gloves off for the main event. The winners and still champions are you and Controlled Cheating. "Happy Day Is Here Again." You can eat *anything* and *everything* and *as much as you want.* All the Diet Derbies, guilts, and hungers are forgotten for today. Your unused teeth are ready for action.

On the mornings of my Controlled Cheating Days, I wake up with the birds and sing like a nasal lark. As I lay in bed staring up at my white cottage cheese ceiling, joy shoots through my body and I leap ecstatically straight up.

Skip ahead a few pages and look at the lists of cheating foods. This is my Hit List. You can probably add a few hundred of your own. I've divided them into three fattening categories: dough, sugar, and grease. I think I slapped on a couple of pounds just reading those names. The categories are there to give you a giggle but there is a more serious purpose. Cheating Eating has been my life for nigh on to twenty-two years. In all that time, there's only one piece of wisdom I've learned:

MAKE YOUR CONTROLLED CHEATING DAY SPECIAL

When I talk about making your Cheating Day special, I'm telling you to plan your menu in advance. But it's okay to deviate. Suppose you're strolling by a store that day and you get a crazy craving for macadamia nut brittle. Great. Add it on.

Planning ahead means cheating with the foods you truly, deeply love. It's really very romantic. Don't waste calories on any old food because it's there. Eat your heart's desire to your heart's content, but do it with love. Enjoy, savor, and eat your goodies slowly.

At the end of the big day, as you're slumped in the recliner full and happy, you'll be able to look back over the day with satisfaction and affection. You won't think back and moan, my God, why did I eat that stupid white gummy roll with margarine.

Another biggie is that you should not use up valuable calories and space in the stomach department with foods that you are only lukewarm about. Be red hot about everything you gorge on.

Again though, this is *your* fun day. You can eat your way through the Dolly Madison Cake Plant or you can have five fettucinis in forty minutes or you can walk around your favorite enclosed mall going from Dairy Queen to Taco Bell to Topsy's Popcorn to Kentucky Fried.

My calculator and I have figured out the calories and portion sizes for the Hit List. This is not so you can pass out if you add up the calories you glommed on a Cheating Eating Day. It's just to let you know what you're doing even on Controlled Cheating Days and every step of your slim life.

What you are going to find directly ahead are seven sample Controlled Cheating Days. This is to give you an idea of how you can construct a full day's valuable eating. It is not necessary to follow any of these menus exactly; after these seven samples are long lists of goodies which you can put together in any way that suits your fancy, tickles your palate, and—sob, sob—flattens your wallet.

GREASED LIGHTNING

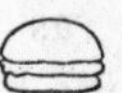

A Fast-Food Fantasy

BREAKFAST AT MCDONALD'S	CALORIES
Egg McMuffin	350
Hash brown potatoes	130
Hot chocolate	160
MID-MORNING SNACK AT DUNKIN' DONUTS	
One glazed doughnut	170
LUNCH AT ARTHUR TREACHER'S FISH AND CHIPS	
Fish (2 pieces)	355
Chips	275
MID-AFTERNOON SNACK AT DAIRY QUEEN	
Ice cream cone, plain large	340
DINNER AT KENTUCKY FRIED CHICKEN	
Original recipe chicken, Dinner One (wing and rib)	604
Potatoes and gravy	84
Coleslaw	122
Corn	169
Rolls	61

BEDTIME SNACK AT BASKIN-ROBBINS

Ice cream cone—2 scoops (Pralines 'N Cream and French Vanilla)	358
Total Calories	3338

SNACKS, CRACKLE, POP

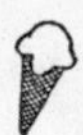

Snacking Only, No Meals In Between

MORNING MUNCH	CALORIES
Kellogg's Pop-Tarts, chocolate frosted	240
Sealtest chocolate milk, 1 glass	205

MID-MORNING MUNCH

Hostess Twinkies, 2 pieces	270
Dad's Root Beer, 6 ounces	80

LUNCH MUNCH

Hot dog on a roll	290
Lay's Potato Chips, 2 ounces	310
Coke, 12 ounces	150

MID-AFTERNOON MUNCH

Pineapple sundae, fountain size	310

EVENING MUNCH

Chili con carne, canned with beans (Hormel), 7½-ounce can	340
Crackers, Krispy Saltines, 10 pieces	100
Shasta Orange Soda, 12 ounces	180

BEDTIME MUNCH

Pecan pie, Home Recipe (USDA), 1 crust, ⅙ of 9-inch pie	575
Vanilla milk shake	310
TOTAL CALORIES	3245

STAND AND DRIP

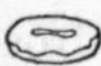

Non-Seating Eating—You Can Take It with You

BREAKFAST	CALORIES
Pepperidge Farm Apple Strudel, ⅙	205

MID-MORNING SNACK

Dutch Apple Dannon Yogurt, 1 container	260

LUNCH

Burger King Double Meat Whopper with cheese	950

Onion rings	270
Vanilla shake	340

MID-AFTERNOON SNACK

7-Up, 12 ounces	150

DINNER

Pizza Hut, Thin 'N Crispy cheese pizza, 2 slices	340
Canada Dry ginger ale, 12 ounces	130
Chips Ahoy, 5 cookies	275

BEDTIME SNACK

Cracker Jacks, 3-ounce box	350
TOTAL CALORIES	3270

ALL AMERICAN DAY

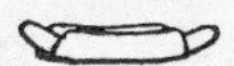

Star Spangled Eating

BREAKFAST	CALORIES
Aunt Jemima pancake mix, 3 (4-inch) cakes with syrup,	
4 tablespoons Log Cabin,	
1 tablespoon butter	480
3 slices fried bacon	135

MID-MORNING SNACK

Corn muffin, 1 piece, 1 tablespoon Smucker's preserves, any flavor	235

LUNCH

McDonald's Big Mac	540
French fries	210
Chocolate shake	360

MID-AFTERNOON SNACK

Frozen Milky Way	120

DINNER

1 pound sirloin steak	1316
1 baked potato with sour cream	225
Coca-Cola, 12 ounces	150
Homemade apple pie, 1/6 of a 9-inch pie with 1/4 pint vanilla ice cream	555

BEDTIME SNACK

Planters cocktail oil roasted peanuts, 1 ounce	185
TOTAL CALORIES	3956

JUST DESSERTS

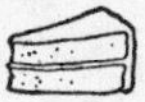

The Sweetest Day of Your Life

BREAKFAST	CALORIES
Aunt Jemima frozen waffle with syrup, 1 double waffle as packaged, 1 tablespoon butter	265
Hydrox Cookies, 6 cookies	300
MID-MORNING SNACK	
Keebler Coconut Bars, 4 bars	240
LUNCH	
Banana cream pie, Banquet frozen, ⅓ of pie	350
1 glass Birds Eye Lemonade	100
MID-AFTERNOON SNACK	
Chocolate eclair, custard filled	315
DINNER	
Sara Lee frozen cream cheese cake, 1 whole cake	855
BEDTIME SNACK	
Hostess Ding Dong, 1 piece	170
Milk shake, any flavor	310

OPTIONAL

24 glasses of tap water	000
Total Calories	2835

SUPERMARKET SCHLEPP

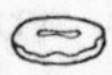

Instant Eats

BREAKFAST	CALORIES
1 water bagel	165
Borden's mozzarella, 1 ounce	95
Hi-C, 1 can	130

MID-MORNING SNACK

Pepperidge Farm Fudge Chip Cookies, 5 cookies	250

LUNCH

2 Wonder bread and Hormel beef bologna sandwiches, 2 ounces bologna on each sandwich with plenty of mustard	640
Dr. Pepper, 12 ounces	140
Keebler pecan fudge brownie, 1 piece	265

MID-AFTERNOON SNACK

Snickers candy bar	130

DINNER

Use additional Wonder bread to make 2 ham and cheese sandwiches	600
Sealtest chocolate milk, individual container	205
Doritos tortilla chips, 2 ounces	180

BEDTIME SNACK

Sealtest strawberry ice cream, 1 pint	520
Total Calories	3320

CLASSIC GOLDBERG

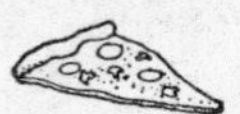

Everything That Doesn't Move

BREAKFAST	CALORIES
French toast, Eggo frozen, 3 slices, with 1 tablespoon butter and 2 tablespoons Log Cabin syrup	440

MID-MORNING SNACK

Morton's Frozen Glazed Donuts, 2	300

LUNCH

Wendy's Triple Cheeseburger	400
French fries	120
Frosty	250

MID-AFTERNOON SNACK

Popcorn, butter and salt added, 6 cups	240
Pepsi-Cola, 12 ounces	160

DINNER

Lasagne, 8 ounces	340
Pepperidge Farm Italian Brown and Serve Bread, 3 slices with 1 tablespoon butter	340
Pepsi-Cola, 12 ounces	160
Fudgsicle	155

BEDTIME SNACK

Payday candy bar	125
TOTAL CALORIES	3030

GREASE, DOUGH, AND SUGAR

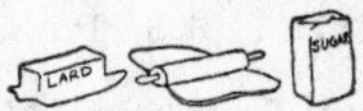

The greatest foods in the world, the ones that are going to enrich your life, fall mainly, as I've said, into one or more of three magnificent categories: grease, dough, and/or sugar.

Some, which I consider super foods, like glazed doughnuts and hot dogs loaded with mustard, fit into all three categories because of the scrumptious nature of their ingredients.

Just like Caesar divided all of Gaul into three parts, so has Julius Caesar Goldberg divided all the treasures of Controlled Cheating Eating into three yummy groups.

Unlike the seven basic food groups we're supposed to eat from daily for a balanced diet, you can hop, skip, and jump back and forth from my groups without a single thought about nutrition to ruin your Cheating Day.

I ate only from grease, dough, and sugar to lift me to my stupendous 325 big ones. But remember that every day of my first twenty-five years was a Cheating Day—and Uncontrolled at that.

Now we're reversing the situation. We're using those three groups not to make you fat, but, in a careful controlled way, to help you lose weight and keep it off. You can believe the Controlled Cheating Diet allows you to enjoy these foods on your special day.

I included portion sizes and calorie counts so you will always know what you are doing, even on a Cheating Day.

These lists are only a sampling from a small group of my all-time favorites. Feel free to cheat with any favorite of yours that I've overlooked. If you have any old family recipes laying around, or regional favorites of dynamite cheating foods, please write immediately with full instructions so I can expand my own cheating horizons.

Cheating Foods with Calorie Counts

COOKIES, 1 PIECE, AS PACKAGED	CALORIES
Animal Crackers (Nabisco Barnum's)	10
Chocolate (Pepperidge Farm Fudge Chip)	50
Chocolate chip (Chips Ahoy!)	55
Coconut (Keebler Bars)	60
Chocolate (Oreo)	50
Chocolate (Hydrox)	50
Fig Newtons	60
Graham crackers, sugar-honey coated (Nabisco)	30
Graham crackers, chocolate covered (Nabisco)	55
Marshmallow, chocolate covered (Mallomars)	60
Lorna Doone	40

	CALORIES
Vanilla (Sunshine Wafers)	15
Pecan Sandies (Keebler)	85

PIES AND PASTRIES

Apple, Home Recipe (USDA), 1/6 of 9-inch pie	405
Apple, frozen (Morton), 1 slice, 1/8 of pie	180
Butterscotch (1 crust), 1/8 of pie	305
Cherry, Home Recipe (USDA), 2 crusts, 1/6 of 9-inch pie	410
Cherry, frozen (Banquet), 1 slice, 1/8 of whole pie	175
Custard (1 crust), 1/8 of whole pie	250
Lemon meringue (1 crust), 1/8 of whole pie	265
Banana cream or Custard, Home Recipe (USDA), 1/6 of 9-inch pie	335

		CALORIES
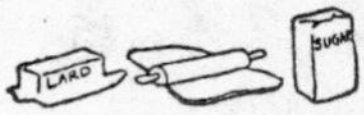	*Banana cream, frozen (Banquet), 1 slice, ⅙ of whole pie*	*175*
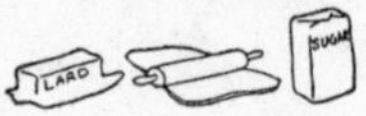	*Boston cream pie, mix (Betty Crocker), ⅛ of pie*	*270*
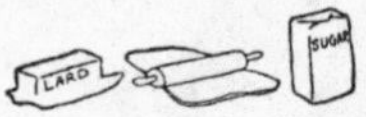	*Chocolate chiffon, Home Recipe (USDA), ⅙ of 9-inch pie*	*460*
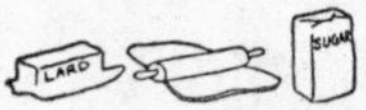	*Chocolate cream, frozen (Morton), 1 slice, ⅙ of 16-ounce pie*	*200*
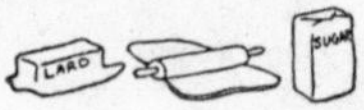	*Mince, frozen (Banquet), ⅙ of 20-ounce pie*	*250*
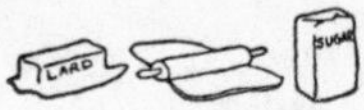	*Mince, Home Recipe (USDA), 2 crusts, ⅙ of 9-inch pie*	*430*
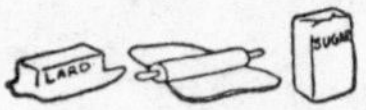	*Pecan, Home Recipe (USDA), 1 crust, ⅙ of 9-inch pie*	*575*
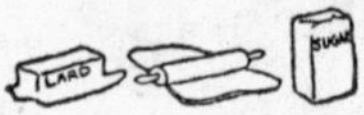	*Pumpkin, Home Recipe (USDA), 1 crust, ⅙ of 9-inch pie*	*320*
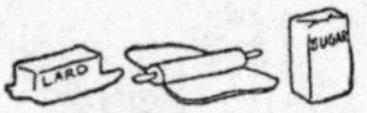	*Pumpkin, frozen (Morton), ⅙ of 24-ounce pie*	*325*
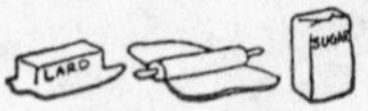	*Apple strudel (Pepperidge Farm), ⅙ of 14-ounce strudel*	*205*

OTHER BAKED GOODIES

	CALORIES
Brownies, pecan fudge (Keebler), 1 brownie as packaged	265
Doughnuts, glazed, frozen (Morton), 1 doughnut as packaged	150
Toaster pastries, all flavors (Toast'Em Pop-Ups), 1¾-ounce	180
Toaster pastries, chocolate, frosted (Kellogg's Pop-Tarts), 1.8-ounce	240

JELLIES AND PRESERVES, 1 TABLESPOON

Jelly, all flavors (Smucker's)	50
Preserves, all flavors (Smucker's)	55

SYRUPS, 1 TABLESPOON

Chocolate flavored (Hershey's)	40
Maple flavored (Log Cabin)	50

DESSERT TOPPINGS, 1 TABLESPOON	CALORIES
Butterscotch (Kraft)	55
Pecans in syrup (Smucker's)	75
Cool Whip, frozen, non-dairy	15
Dream Whip	15

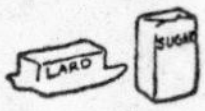

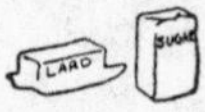

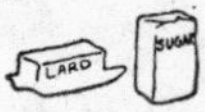

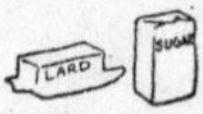

SWEET BAKING INGREDIENTS, 1 OUNCE	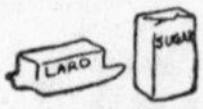
Chocolate semisweet (Nestlé's Morsels)	150
Coconut (Baker's Fine Grated)	150
Sugar, granulated, 1 tablespoon	40

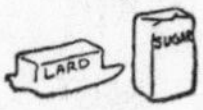

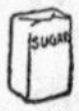

ICE CREAM, ¼ PINT	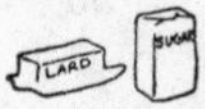
Chocolate (Sealtest)	140
Strawberry (Sealtest)	130
Vanilla (Sealtest), 10.2 percent fat	150

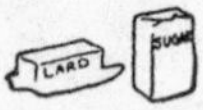

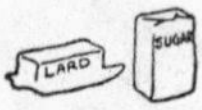

ICE CREAM AND FROZEN GOODIES	CALORIES
Popsicle, 3-fluid-ounce bar	70
Creamsicle, 3-fluid-ounce bar	95
Fudgsicle, 2½-fluid-ounce bar	155
Eskimo Pie ice cream bar, 1 bar	200
Sealtest Ice Cream Sandwich, 1 sandwich	170
Milk shake, most flavors, fountain size	310
Malted milk, most flavors, fountain size	600
Chocolate ice cream soda, 1 scoop, fountain size	300
Pineapple sundae, fountain size	310

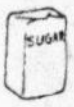

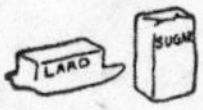

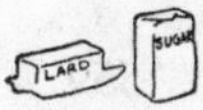

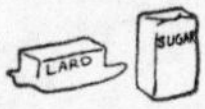

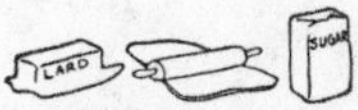

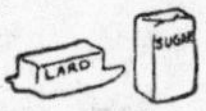

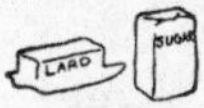

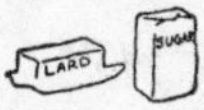

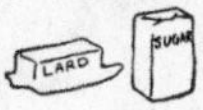

NIBBLES	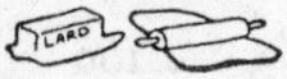
Corn chips (Fritos), 1 ounce	165
Potato chips (Lay's), 1 ounce	155
Potato sticks (Wise), 1 ounce	140

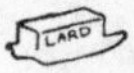

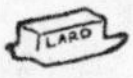

		CALORIES
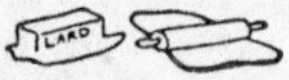	*Tortilla chips (Doritos), 1 ounce*	*140*
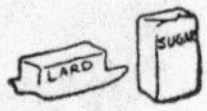	*Peanut butter (Skippy Super Chunk), 1 tablespoon*	*110*
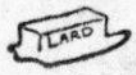	*Blue cheese (Kraft Ready Dip), 8-ounce can*	*550*

NUTS, 1 OUNCE

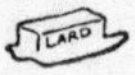	*Almonds (Blue Diamond), barbecued*	*180*
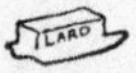	*Brazil (4 nuts)*	*95*
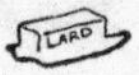	*Cashews (Planters), dry roasted*	*170*
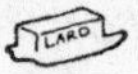	*Cashews (Planters), oil roasted*	*180*
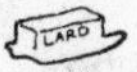	*Coconut, 1 cup shredded*	*450*
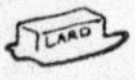	*Chestnuts (6 small)*	*60*
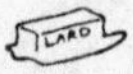	*Mixed (Planters), oil roasted with peanuts*	*185*
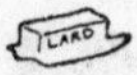	*Peanuts (Skippy), dry roasted*	*180*
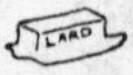	*Peanuts, canned (Planters Cocktail), oil roasted*	*185*
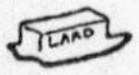	*Pistachios (30 nuts)*	*90*

		CALORIES
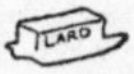	*Pecans (Planters), dry roasted*	205
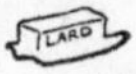	*Walnuts (10 nuts)*	100

POPCORN

	Plain, large kernel (USDA), 1 cup	25
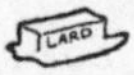	*Butter or oil and salt added (USDA), 1 cup*	40
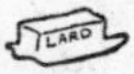	*Butter flavored, ready-to-eat in bags (Wise), 1 cup*	55
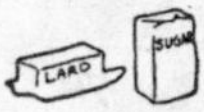	*Cracker Jack, 3-ounce box*	350

PRETZELS

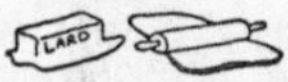

	Pretzel logs (Bachman), 1 piece	20
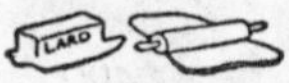	*Mister Salty 3-ring (Nabisco)*	10

SALAD DRESSINGS, 1 TABLESPOON

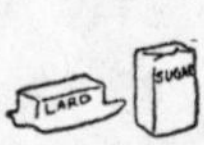

	Blue cheese, bottled (Kraft)	75
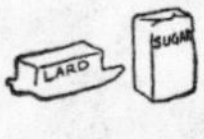	*Caesar, bottled (Seven Seas)*	70
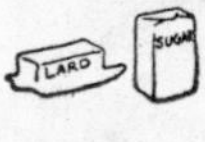	*French, bottled (Kraft)*	65

		CALORIES
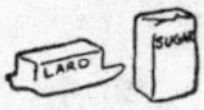	*Green Goddess, bottled (Seven Seas)*	70
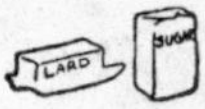	*Italian, bottled (Wishbone)*	80
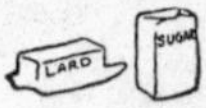	*Mayonnaise, bottled (Hellmann's)*	100
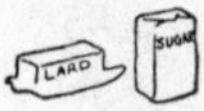	*Roquefort, bottled (Kraft)*	60
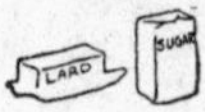	*Russian, bottled (Wishbone)*	55
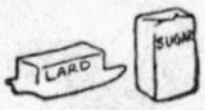	*Thousand Island, bottled (Kraft)*	60
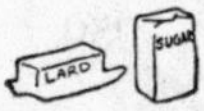	*Miracle Whip, bottled (Kraft)*	70

PUDDINGS, 1 CUP

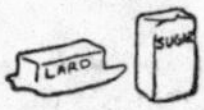	*Butterscotch, instant mix, prepared (Jell-O)*	360
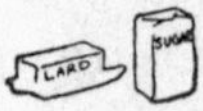	*Chocolate, instant mix, prepared (Royal)*	400
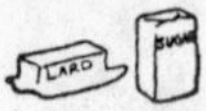	*Lemon, instant mix, prepared (Jell-O)*	360
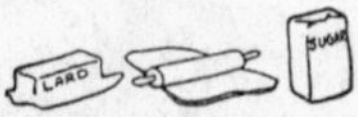	*Bread pudding with raisins, Home Recipe (USDA)*	495
	Gelatin, all flavors, prepared mix (Jell-O), ½ cup	80

CANDY, 1 OUNCE

		CALORIES
SUGAR	*Good and Plenty candy-coated licorice*	100
LARD SUGAR	*Malted milk balls*	130
LARD SUGAR	*Mars bars*	125
LARD SUGAR	*Milky Way*	120
LARD SUGAR	*M & M's, chocolate and peanut*	140
SUGAR	*Campfire Marshmallows*	100
LARD SUGAR	*Welch's Peppermint Patties*	110
LARD SUGAR	*Baby Ruth*	135
LARD SUGAR	*Oh Henry*	130
LARD SUGAR	*Payday*	125
LARD SUGAR	*Powerhouse*	120
LARD SUGAR	*Planter's Peanut Block*	140
LARD SUGAR	*Slo-Poke sucker*	100

		CALORIES
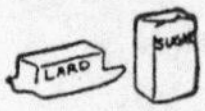	*Snickers*	130
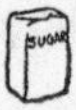	*Tootsie Pops*	150
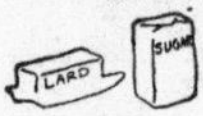	*Tootsie Roll*	115
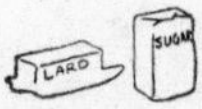	*Hershey Kisses, milk chocolate, 1 piece*	30
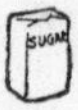	*Life Savers, 1 mint*	5
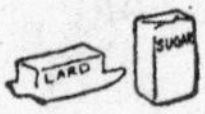	*Reese's Peanut Butter Cup, .6-ounce cup*	90
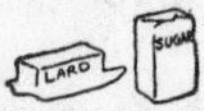	*Butterfinger*	130
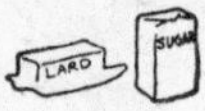	*Chocolate or vanilla caramels (Kraft)*	115
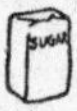	*Chuckles*	90
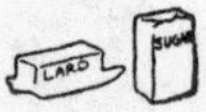	*Sugar Daddy, vanilla*	115
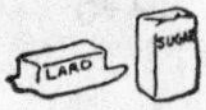	*Milk Duds (Holloway)*	110
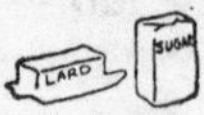	*Hershey Bar, milk chocolate*	150
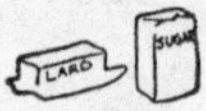	*Hershey Bar, milk chocolate, with almonds*	155
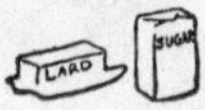	*Chunky, with fruit and nuts*	135

	CALORIES
Nestlé's Crunch, chocolate crunch bar	150
Mounds	125
Almond Joy	130
Reed's hard candies, all flavors	110
Mason Dots jellied candy	100
Black Crows licorice	100
Red Hot Dollars	95

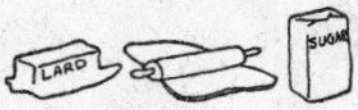

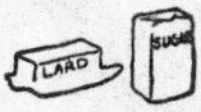

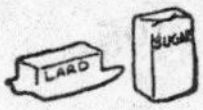

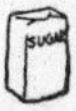

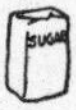

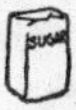

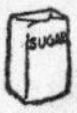

CAKES

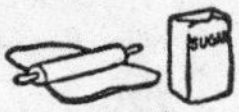

Angel food, Home Recipe (USDA), 1/12 of an 8-inch cake	110
Banana, frozen (Sara Lee), 1/8 of cake	175
Cheesecake, frozen, cream cheese (Sara Lee), 1/3 of cake	285
Chocolate, Home Recipe (USDA), with chocolate icing, 2-layer, 1/12 of a 9-inch cake	365

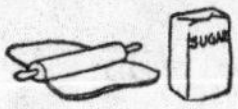

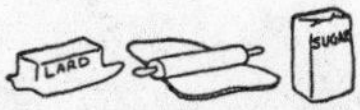

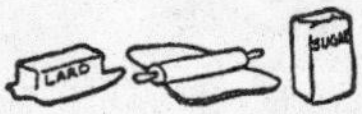

		CALORIES
	Chocolate, frozen (Pepperidge Farm), 1/6 of cake	*315*
	Coffee cake, frozen (Sara Lee), pecan, large, 1/8 of cake	*165*
	Devil's food, frozen (Sara Lee), 1/8 of cake	*190*
	Gingerbread, 1/9 of an 8-inch square	*175*
	Pound cake, frozen (Sara Lee), regular, 1/10 of cake	*125*
	Cupcake with chocolate icing, 2½ inches	*130*

SNACK CAKES

	Chocolate-coated Ding Dongs (Hostess), 1 (3/8-ounce) cake	*170*
	Twinkies (Hostess), 1 (3/8-ounce) cake	*135*
	Eclair, custard filling, chocolate icing	*315*
	Doughnut, plain	*125*

MILK DRINKS	CALORIES
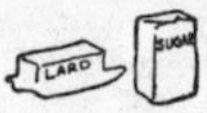 *Chocolate milk (Sealtest), 3.5 percent butterfat, dairy packed, 8-ounce glass*	205
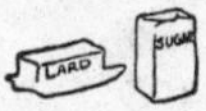 *Chocolate mix, prepared (Hershey's Hot Chocolate), 1 ounce in 8-ounce glass of whole milk*	275

CREAM, 1 TABLESPOON

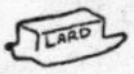 *Half and half, 12 percent butterfat (Sealtest)*	20
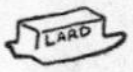 *Heavy, whipping (Foremost)*	55

YOGURT, 8-OUNCE CUP

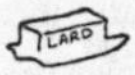 *Plain (Dannon)*	130
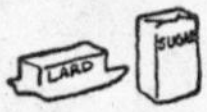 *Strawberry (Dannon)*	260

CHEESE AND CHEESE PRODUCTS, 1 OUNCE

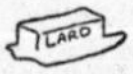 *American (Kraft)*	105
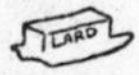 *Camembert (Borden's)*	85
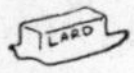 *Gruyére (Kraft)*	110
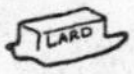 *Mozzarella (Borden's)*	95

	CALORIES
Muenster (Kraft)	*100*
Parmesan (Kraft)	*105*
Pizza (Borden's)	*85*
Roquefort (Kraft)	*105*
Swiss (Dorman's Endeco)	*90*
Cream cheese (Kraft Philadelphia)	*105*
Cheez Whiz	*75*
Velveeta	*85*

STEAK

Porterhouse steak, 1 pound, broiled, lean and fat, yield after cooking 10.6 ounces	*1,400*
Sirloin steak, 1 pound, broiled, lean and fat, yield after cooking 10.9 ounces	*1,192*

BREAD, 1 SLICE ONLY, CHEATER

Date Nut (Thomas')	*90*
Italian, brown and serve, baked (Pepperidge Farm)	*80*

		CALORIES
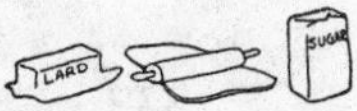	*Cinnamon-raisin (Pepperidge Farm)*	*75*

BREADSTICKS, 1 STICK

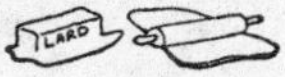

	Plain (Stella D'Oro)	*40*

MUFFINS AND ROLLS, 1 PIECE

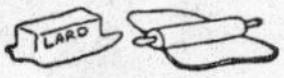

	Biscuits, refrigerator, buttermilk, baked (Pillsbury)	*105*
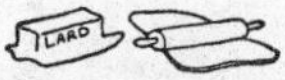	*Corn (Thomas')*	*180*
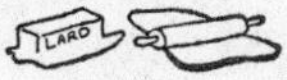	*Frankfurter roll (Wonder), 2-ounce bun*	*160*
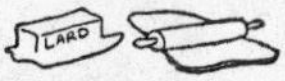	*English (Thomas')*	*140*
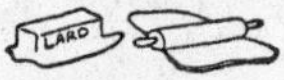	*Hard roll, brown and serve, baked (Pepperidge Farm Club)*	*120*
	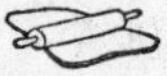 *Bagel, water (USDA), 3-inch*	*165*

CRACKERS, 1 PIECE AS PACKAGED

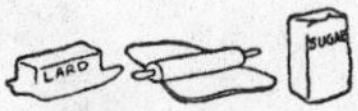

	Bacon flavored (Nabisco Bacon Thins)	*10*
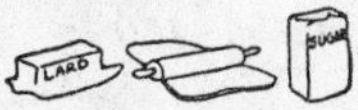	*Ritz Cracker*	*20*
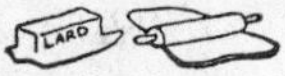	*Cheez-It Cracker*	*5*

	CALORIES
Matzo, 1 sheet (Manischewitz regular)	110
Saltine (Krispy)	10

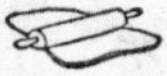

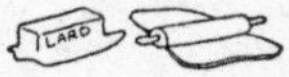

PANCAKES AND WAFFLES

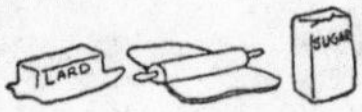

Pancake, plain, Home Recipe (USDA), 4-inch pancake, prepared with egg and milk	60
Waffle, Home Recipe (USDA), 7-inch waffle	210
Pancake mix, prepared (Aunt Jemima), 4-inch cake, made according to package directions	60
Waffle, frozen (Aunt Jemima), 1 double waffle as packaged	115
Waffle mix, prepared (Aunt Jemima Easy Pour), 4½-inch waffle	190
French toast, frozen (Eggo), 1 slice	80

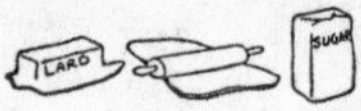

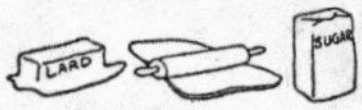

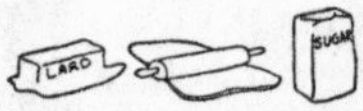

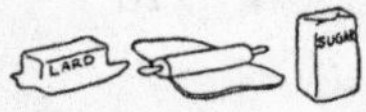

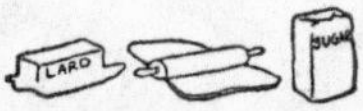

SODA, 12-OUNCE GLASS

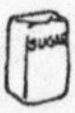

Coca-Cola	150
Pepsi-Cola	160

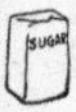

		CALORIES
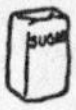	*Dr. Pepper*	*140*
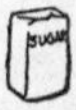	*Royal Crown*	*160*
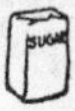	*Dr. Brown cream soda*	*170*
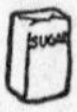	*Canada Dry ginger ale*	*140*
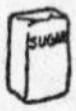	*Shasta orange soda*	*180*
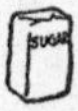	*Dad's Root Beer*	*160*
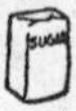	*7-Up*	*150*

ASSORTED DRINKS

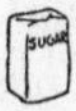	*Kool-Aid, all flavors, fruit, mix, prepared*	*95*
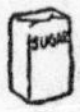	*Lemonade, frozen (Birds Eye), reconstituted, 8-ounce glass*	*100*
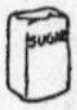	*Punch, canned (Hi-C)*	*130*

POTATOES

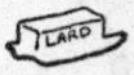	*French-fried in deep fat (USDA), 10 pieces*	*155*

		CALORIES
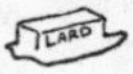	*French-fried, frozen (Ore-Ida Golden Crinkles), 17 pieces*	100
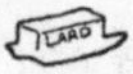	*Mashed mix, prepared (Betty Crocker Potato Buds), made according to package, ⅓ of cup*	135
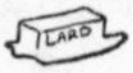	*Potato salad, Home Recipe (USDA), with mayonnaise and French dressing, hard-cooked eggs, seasonings, 4 ounces*	165

BAKED BEANS

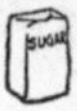	*Baked beans in tomato sauce (Heinz), ½ cup*	135
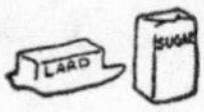	*Baked beans with pork in tomato sauce (Heinz), ½ cup*	150

ALL SORTS OF CHEATING EATING FOODS

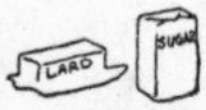	*Frankfurter, all beef (Oscar Mayer), 1.6 ounces*	140
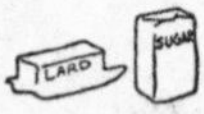	*Ham, cured (Swift Boneless), 4 ounces*	190
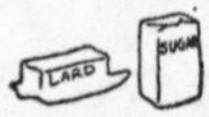	*Corned beef, canned (Armour Star), 4 ounces*	320
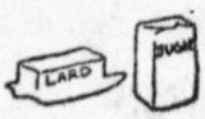	*Sloppy Joe, canned (Libby's) beef, ¼ of 15¼-ounce can*	175

		CALORIES
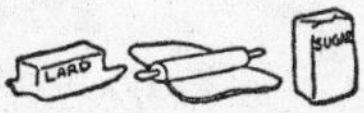	*Chicken pot pie, frozen (Swanson), 8 ounces*	505
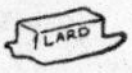	*Sardines, in oil, drained (King Oscar), 3¾-ounce can*	170
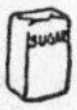	*Shrimp, with cocktail sauce (Sau-Sea), 6-ounce jar*	120
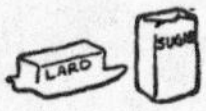	*Bacon, medium sliced (USDA), 1 slice broiled or fried crisp*	45
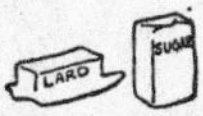	*Bacon, Canadian style (USDA), 1-ounce slice broiled or fried crisp*	80
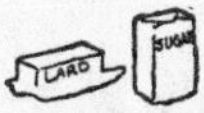	*Bologna, pure beef (Hormel), 1 ounce*	85
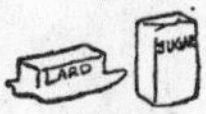	*Salami, pure beef (Oscar Mayer), 1 slice*	40
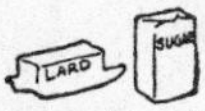	*Link sausage, smokie (Oscar Mayer), 1.5-ounce link*	135
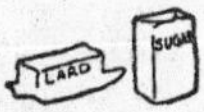	*Chow mein, chicken, canned without noodles (Chun King), 1 cup*	75
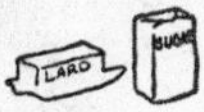	*Chili con carne, canned without beans (Hormel), ½ of a 15-ounce can*	340
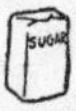	*Chili con carne, canned with beans (Hormel), 7½-ounce can*	320

		CALORIES
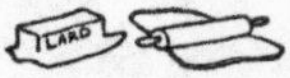	*Tamales, jar or can (Armour Star), 1 tamale*	90
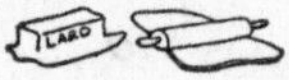	*Tortillas, canned (Old El Paso), 1 tortilla*	40

FROZEN DINNERS, 1 COMPLETE DINNER

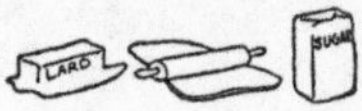	*Beans and Franks (Banquet), 10¾ ounces*	590
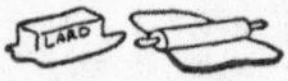	*Fried Chicken (Banquet), 11 ounces*	540
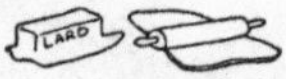	*Macaroni and Cheese (Morton), 11 ounces*	335
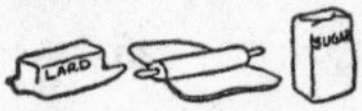	*Spaghetti and Meatballs (Banquet), 11½ ounces*	425
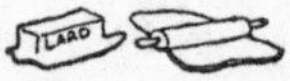	*Chop Suey Beef Dinner (Banquet), 12 ounces*	280

PASTA, COOKED

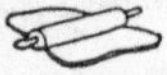	*Egg noodles, all varieties (Ronzoni), 1 cup*	200
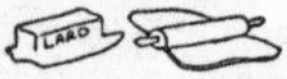	*Macaroni, all varieties (Goodman's), 1 cup*	150
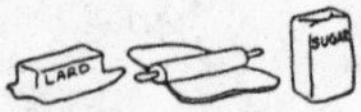	*Spaghetti, all varieties (Buitoni), 1 cup*	165
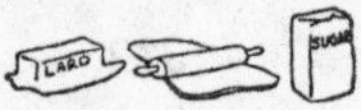	*Spaghetti with meatballs and tomato sauce, canned (SpaghettiO's), 1 cup*	230

		CALORIES
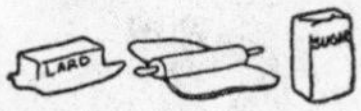	*Lasagne, frozen (Buitoni), 8 ounces*	340
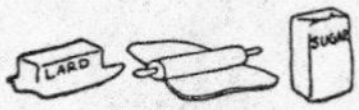	*Ravioli, with meat and sauce (Buitoni), 8 ounces*	280

FATS

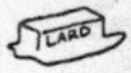	*Butter (USDA), 1 tablespoon*	100
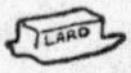	*Margarine (Parkay), 1 tablespoon*	100
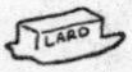	*Shortening (Crisco), 1 tablespoon*	105

SANDWICHES

Okay, Controlled Cheaters, the calories for these sandwiches are approximations depending on how much stuff you load on the bread. These calories are *not* for sandwiches that you play like Dagwood Bumstead.

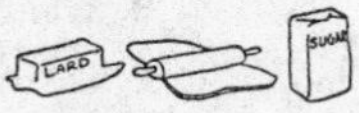	*Frankfurter*	290
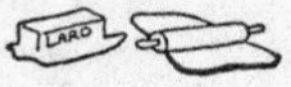	*Hamburger*	310
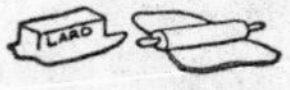	*Cheeseburger*	410
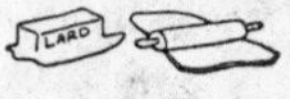	*Roast beef*	375
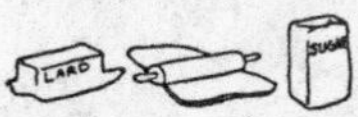	*Bacon, lettuce, and tomato*	275
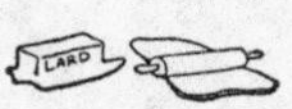	*Smoked salmon with cream cheese on a bagel*	325

	CALORIES
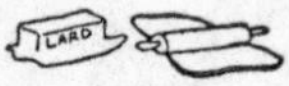 *Meatloaf*	300
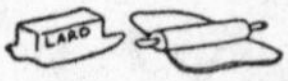 *Sliced chicken*	220
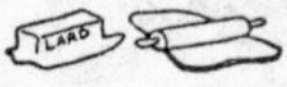 *Chicken salad*	325
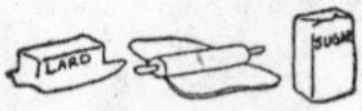 *Peanut butter and jelly*	345
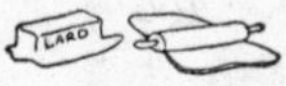 *Cheese and sliced tomato*	280
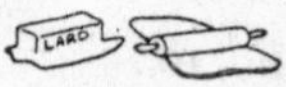 *Chopped chicken liver*	275
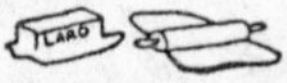 *Liverwurst*	310
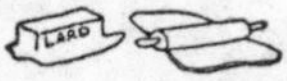 *Club*	415
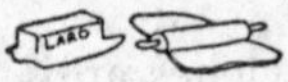 *Egg salad*	335
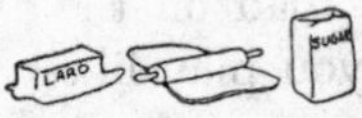 *Ham and cheese*	300
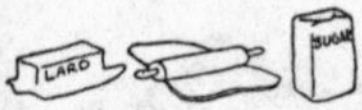 *Boiled ham*	265
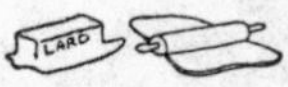 *Tuna salad*	225

PIZZA

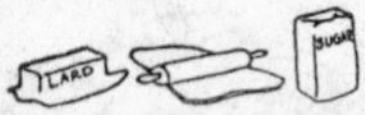 *Cheese, frozen (Celeste), ½ of 7-ounce pie*	245
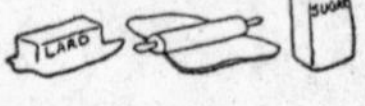 *Sausage, frozen (Jenos), ½ of 13½-ounce pie*	450

	CALORIES
Pepperoni, frozen (Celeste), ½ of a 7½-ounce pie	*265*
Deluxe, frozen (Celeste), ½ of a 9-inch pie	*300*

FAST-FOOD CALORIE COUNTS

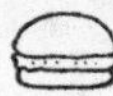

I've always lived life in the fast-food lane. My folks should have named me Burger Kingberg. As I've learned over the years, across their counters and under their Golden Arches, these are the hot spots I've known and loved desperately. Now I feel you should know how many glorious calories you're munching at each stop. I've spared no time, effort, and expense in researching this info. "I did it all for You, you're the one!"

Pizza Hut

2 slices of a medium pizza

THIN 'N' CRISPY	CALORIES
Standard cheese	340
Super-style cheese	410
Standard pepperoni	370
Super-style pepperoni	430
Standard pork and mushroom	380

Super-style pork and mushroom	450
Supreme	400
Super-supreme	520

THICK 'N' CHEWY

Standard cheese	390
Super-style cheese	450
Standard pepperoni	450
Super-style pepperoni	490
Standard pork and mushroom	430
Super-style pork and mushroom	500
Supreme	480
Super-supreme	590

McDonald's

	CALORIES
Hamburger	260
Cheeseburger	300
Quarter Pounder Hamburger	420
Quarter Pounder with Cheese	520
Big Mac	540
Filet-O-Fish	400
Egg McMuffin	350
Hotcakes with syrup/butter	470
Scrambled eggs	160
Sausage	180
English muffin	190
Hash brown potatoes	130
French fries	210

Hot chocolate	160
Chocolate shake	360
Strawberry shake	340
Vanilla shake	320
Apple pie	300
Cherry pie	300
McDonaldland cookies	290
Hot fudge sundae	290
Caramel sundae	290
Strawberry sundae	230
Pineapple sundae	230

Baskin-Robbins Ice Cream

All calories are for one scoop of ice cream

	CALORIES
Vanilla ice cream	147
Chocolate ice cream	165
Strawberry ice cream	141
French vanilla ice cream	181
Chocolate fudge ice cream	178
Pralines 'n' cream ice cream	177
Orange sherbet	99
Daiquiri ice	84

Kentucky Fried Chicken

ORIGINAL RECIPE CHICKEN

	CALORIES
Dinner 1	
Wing and Rib	604

Dinner 2	
Wing and Thigh	662
Dinner 3	
Drumstick and Thigh	643

EXTRA CRISPY CHICKEN

Dinner 1	
Wing and Rib	755
Dinner 2	
Wing and Thigh	812
Dinner 3	
Drumstick and Thigh	765

ORIGINAL RECIPE CHICKEN

Wing	136
Drumstick	117
Rib	199
Thigh	257
Keel	236

EXTRA CRISPY CHICKEN

Wing	201
Drumstick	155
Rib	286
Thigh	343
Keel	297

SIDE ITEMS

Potatoes	63
Gravy	23

Coleslaw	122
Rolls	61
Corn	169

Wendy's

	CALORIES
Single hamburger	200
Double hamburger	285
Triple hamburger	360
Single cheeseburger	240
Double cheeseburger	325
Triple cheeseburger	400
Chili	250
French fries	120
Frosty	250

Arthur Treacher's Fish and Chips

	CALORIES
Chowder	110
Fish (2 pieces)	355
Chicken (2 pieces)	370
Shrimp (7 pieces)	380
Krunch Pup	205
Fish sandwich	440
Chicken sandwich	415

Chips	275
Coleslaw	125
Lemon Luv	275

Burger King

	CALORIES
Hamburger	295
Hamburger with Cheese	345
Doublemeat Hamburger	415
Doublemeat Hamburger with Cheese	520
Whopper Jr.	370
Whopper Jr. with Cheese	425
Whopper Jr. Doublemeat	490
Whopper Jr. Doublemeat with Cheese	545
Whopper	630
Whopper with Cheese	740
Whopper Doublemeat	845
Whopper Doublemeat with Cheese	950
French fries	
Regular	210
Large	360
Onion rings	
Regular	265
Large	330
Vanilla shake	335
Chocolate shake	335
Apple pie	250

Dairy Queen

	CALORIES
Hamburgers	
Single	370
Single with Cheese	470
Double	540
Double with Cheese	650
Triple	740
Triple with Cheese	840
Fish Sandwich	400
Fish Sandwich with Cheese	440
French fries	
2.5 ounces	200
4.0 ounces	320
Onion rings	300
Plain Cone	
Small	110
Medium	230
Large	340
Chocolate Dipped Cone	
Small	150
Medium	300
Large	450
Buster Bar	390
Dilly Bar	240
Banana Split	540
Chocolate Malt	
Small	340
Medium	600
Large	840

Chocolate Sundae	
Small	170
Medium	300
Large	400
Parfait	460
Float	330
Freeze	520
Sandwich	140
Hot Fudge Brownie Delight	570
Mr. Misty Float	440
Mr. Misty Freeze	500

Dunkin' Donuts

	CALORIES
Yeast-raised doughnuts (For glaze, add 5 to 10 calories) (For topping and filling combined, add 40 to 50 calories)	160
Cake and chocolate cake doughnuts (Includes crullers, rings, sticks)	240
Munchkins Yeast-raised	25
Cake and chocolate cake (For topping and filling combined, add 10 to 15 calories)	65
Fancy Stuff (Includes danish, coffee rolls etc.)	215

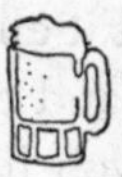

The Day After Your Controlled Cheating Day

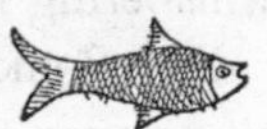

Welcome back. Had a good time? You don't want to come back? You want to keep cheating? Sure, I can understand that. Life was so terrific yesterday. You ate everything you wanted. You felt full and good. Wining, dining, running, and funning around. All those screaming fat cells finally quieted down for a while.

These next twenty-four hours are so important that I'm taking a whole chapter to bring your strawberry balloon back to earth. This is the most crucial, critical, twitchy day in your diet life. Hold on. I don't want to lose you. We both need all the company and help we can get.

Now you're back down to earth. Yesterday went so fast. All your taste buds got into a tizzy with all that action. Everything tasted so good. Many foods your taster had almost forgotten. But didn't those Cheating Eating foods taste ten times better? You hadn't eaten any of those goodies for two weeks. Didn't that make your Controlled Cheating Day even more fun? Absence makes the tummy grow fonder.

Now don't roll over and bury your face in the pillow and start sobbing and beating your little fists against the injustice of it all.

Forget it. You've got to exercise your tough discipline and exorcise your food demons. After a Cheating Eating Day, you feel caught in a velvet vise. They've got you "in between the devil's food cake and the deep dish blueberry pie."

I know those food demons are prancing back and forth on your down-filled comforter and running up and down the walls and ceiling grinning with their lime-flavored Life Saver teeth. Some of your tempting, delicious pals are beckoning, taunting, and whispering in your pearly ears: "Come with us for just another day. Remember those buttery hash brown potatoes? So what if you can't button your mackinaw, you sweat all the time, and your bowling score should be as high as your blood pressure. We've been friends for years. We need you, buddy, more than one day a week. What do ya say, Plumperoo?"

Shut your eyes and scream, "Out, out, damn demons. Be gone. I want no further truck with you for six full days. I shall remember you often, all of you, for we shall meet again in six short days. Who can forget the wonderful times we had yesterday? I'm already planning which ones of you I'm going to be seeing next week on that GREAT COME AND GET IT DAY."

YOUR KNIFE AND FORK PRISON

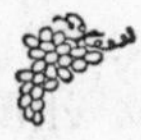

This is the day after your Controlled Cheating Day and you must sentence yourself to go back to the Knife and Fork Prison.

This Slimmer Slammer is a maximum security jail for hardened fatties, located on an island paradise in your mind (next to the Statue of Liberty, that beautiful lady who represents your

Cheating Day). It's a Big House from which you parole yourself once a week. You've sentenced yourself there because you're the judge, jury, warden, guard, and trusty of your slim body.

There are no handcuffs and no solitary confinement, unless you try to break out. Edward G. Robinson, James Cagney, and George Raft won't sneak around and force-feed you pecan waffles with whipped butter and real maple syrup.

On the day after your Controlled Cheating Day, slap on your best slammer smile, pull on your form-fitting striped overalls, and calmly step behind the bars. (No whimpering allowed.) You can have visitors but under no circumstances is there to be a Sara Lee German Chocolate Cake hidden in a file.

Confined in your Knife and Fork Prison there are criminal activities you must give up. You can't hold up a Baskin-Robbins for a pralines and cream cone or saw through a Big Mac with your teeth and expect to get away with it.

Buck up. The prison cafeteria has plenty for you to eat. You won't be on bread and water. You've got your 14-Day Diet Program with hundreds of good food substitutions. As you're sitting behind bars peering out into the free eating world, don't despair; you're going to get sprung in a few days.

Keep staring at the Controlled Cheater's gorgeous heroine, The Statue of Liberty. Your day will come.

FATS GOLDBERG'S DIET DAY EXERCISES FOR TEETH, GUMS, TONGUE, LIPS, CHEEKS, AND JAWS

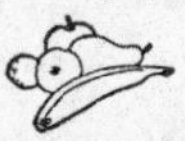

These are specially designed exercises for Controlled Cheaters to use on Diet Days. Since you will not be strenuously using these six vitally important areas of your eating equipment every day, it is imperative that they not get flabby or let spider webs form from their being underused.

You can exercise any time or place. I would advise, however, that you do not exercise in public places because of other folks' severe questioning of your mental capabilities.

Toothpick Tussle: Ram a round or flat toothpick between each tooth. Whirl toothpick four revolutions to the right, then six revolutions to the left or until you take off like a helicopter. If you are wealthy, you may use Stim-U-Dents, Interdental Stimulators.

Molar Mash: This is an isometric exercise. Slowly close molars on a small log like Fido fetching a stick. Wag your tail, sit up, and beg for a treat. (But you can't have it 'til your Cheating Day!)

Dental Floss Slide with Jaw Manipulation: Open jaw wide enough to get unrestricted view of tonsils. Slide unwaxed dental floss between each tooth. If anything interesting comes out, like orange pulp or spinach sprigs, be sure to save it for a snack later on.

Cheeks and Lips Lift: Pucker lips and suck cheeks toward teeth like you are slurping a vanilla malted through a straw. Make loud, rude, inhaling sounds. This will come in handy if you are trying to dry off your teeth or vacuuming the rug.

cheated one dirty, dumb, rotten day and you put back on three quarters of the weight you've struggled to take off.

Never you fret. These gloomy thoughts will soon go away and so will the added weight. I'll tell you how to get rid of both.

1. Surprise, surprise. You didn't really gain back all those tough pounds you've lost. Even *you* can't eat that much. Here you are, after that wonderful Cheating Eating Day and you're still way ahead in the weight-loss game, because you have six more days to lose those Cheating Day pounds and *even* more. So relax.

2. Controlled Cheating is a lifetime plan. You knew you were going to cheat, basically what you were going to eat that day, and probably how much. This is not a two-week diet you crash on and then go bozo and slap all the weight back on. This is an eating program to follow the rest of your skinny days. It takes time. You have time. So relax.

3. You have a dynamite, low-calorie, balanced diet to return to with all sorts of different foods to help you lose the pounds you've added back and then some. So relax.

4. As soon as you can get your eyes unglued from the scale, think back over yesterday, reliving every delicious bite and the hot time you had. Start from the moment your eyes flew open in the morning until you closed your food-heavy lids at night. So relax.

5. While your toes are still curled around the edge of the scale with terror, start thinking about your next Cheating Eating, only six short days away. This is not the end of your eating career, but the beginning. So relax.

As I'm sitting here typing on a beautiful June morning, the tears are falling down my cheeks. Yesterday was a Cheating Day for me, and today when I hopped on my Health-O-Meter, the few remaining hairs on my head stood on end. I had gained six

TIPPING THE SCALES

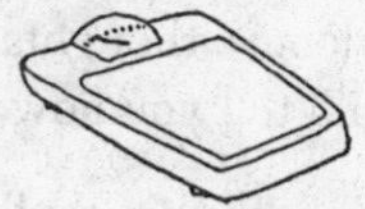

After you brush your teeth, take off all your clothes and pul your pal, the scale, out of its place of honor in the back of the closet and set it on the favorite spot where you always weigh less. Jaunty-jolly step right up on the scale.

Before looking at the dial, smile as wide as you can until the corners of your mouth are almost in your ear drums. Then with courage and mighty resolve, force your baby blues to look down and check where the needle stops. Whatever you do, do not scream out loud. Also, make sure your eyeballs don't fall out from surprise.

Many times after a Cheating Day, I think my eyes are playing tricks on me and I'm not reading the numbers right. I also stand on the scale longer, staring down to make absolutely sure the stupid scale is right. There are days I've almost missed lunch because my feet have been planted on the scale for such a long time. Then I think something is drastically wrong with the scale. THAT NUMBER COULDN'T BE RIGHT! After sticking my head under a cold shower, I become rational again.

You are, of course, going to see a weight gain. Maybe anywhere from one to six pounds, depending on how fast you could stuff it in.

You are going to feel lousy, frustrated, depressed, and you're going to want to throw your Controlled Cheating Diet, your scale, and me out of the window. You might even want to throw yourself after us. Hold on to the shower curtain for moral support if you get too close to the window. These are natural feelings. Who wouldn't get twitchy? You stuck to your diet like Elmer's Glue. You lost plenty of weight and then you went out and pounds. Usually I can tell approximately how much I'm going to gain but I sure got fooled this time.

Sadness and anger poured out of every pore. Then I went through the Fabulous Five Feel-goods I just listed for you and now I feel better. Thanks.

YOU MUST GO BACK ON YOUR DIET

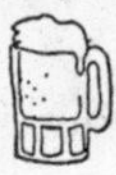

There is absolutely no other way I can say it. I'm looking you straight in the eye and I'm telling you, straight from the shoulder, the truth.

YOU: That is Y-O-U. I'm saying *you*. Not the lady with the Sears shopping bag sitting next to you on the bus, or Ralph down the street, who's having a garage sale, or the husband of your Aunt Hilda. I'm talking to YOU.

MUST: That is M-U-S-T. No maybes, perhapses, or possiblies. MUST means there is no room for maneuvers or delays or tricks you've been playing on yourself. MUST is a command.

GO: G-O means to move. Move to your diet as described in the chapter "Born to Lose." Not sideways or at an angle. That's a straight line to your low-calorie, balanced diet. I'm waiting.

BACK: B-A-C-K means to *return* to the program, to the diet program that you used the last two weeks. You are returning, but at the same time what you are actually doing is moving forward. You are moving forward because you will begin losing weight again and continuing your march to your Goal Weight. BACK, in this case, means full speed ahead.

ON: O-N means following the diet to the letter. You are ON top of the diet. Not underneath, or on the sides, or around the back where you can cheat.

YOUR: Y-O-U-R is the possessive form of you. This is YOUR diet and it's going to give you the form you want to possess. No one is going to knock on your door and tell you they can lose the weight for you. No one else can lose weight and keep it off for you.

DIET: D-I-E-T means the specific weight-loss program outlined for you.

Spelling it out once more for you kids in the back row:

Y-O-U M-U-S-T G-O B-A-C-K O-N Y-O-U-R D-I-E-T!

HARK! LOOK! LISTEN! HEAR YE! HEAR YE!

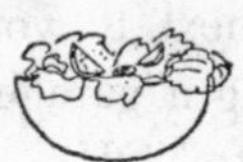

The A Number One accomplishment of my twenty-two years of losing weight and keeping it off is the ability to go back on my diet immediately, the very day after a Controlled Cheating Day.

I know, I know. You're sick of this one thought but I have to keep coming back to it for your sake and mine. *There are no secrets to losing weight and keeping it off*. You'd better get used to this idea because I'm going to come back to it many more times.

If there is one idea, thought, practice, or method that comes close to magic in controlling weight, this is it—the ability to go back on your diet after a Controlled Cheating Day.

Controlled Cheating's success is based on this one principle. This is the guiding light, the royal flush, and the big payoff. The one reason why I have been successful in losing weight (and you can be, too) is my ability to go back, without hemming and hawing or hesitation on the diet after I've cheated. Nothing else counts.

Controlled Cheating is the release. Going back on the diet is the "key." Sometimes the key is hard to turn and you have to force it, but the door that opens is your Open Sesame to slim freedom and happiness.

From my earliest memories, I've been obsessed with losing weight and dieting. I bought every diet book published and went to the best diet doctors in Kansas City. I talked to friends and enemies alike. I cussed. I screamed. I prayed. I tore at my clothes. Finally some kind soul would throw a bucket of cold Pepsi-Cola on me and I returned to reality. And trying to find another diet that would work. That was my reality, my avocation, my full-time job. It was also the beginning of my suspicion of so-called professionals who are supposed to be able to help us. I was finding out how little they really know about obesity.

The saga, pre-age twenty-five, was always the same. I would get every doctor's diet, diet book diet, or a diet from a passing bus driver. I would go on the dumb diet, stick to it for a few days, or maybe even a week or two, then I would cheat one day. It didn't have to be one full day. If I just ate three cinnamon rolls in two minutes, I was gone again. The diet was busted and I rolled out eating faster and harder than ever.

This went on for years. The same vicious cycle. I would start dieting, cheat for one minute, and be off and stuffing it in nonstop for another four months.

In 1957, I was waiting tables at my fraternity house, Zeta Beta Tau, at the University of Missouri. I waited tables because I could eat all I wanted. One lunch I'll never forget: three complete lunches which totaled six greasy cheeseburgers, a gallon of cold applesauce, and a pound of potato chips, plus four chunky peanut butter-and-jelly sandwiches loaded with margarine, two quarts of milk, and three pieces of chocolate cake.

Struggling up the steps from the kitchen, I thought the end

was near. I willed my size 50 khaki pants to Dumbo the elephant. I had been stuffed before but nothing ever like this. Lying down on the floor, out of breath and moaning, a fraternity brother took pity on me and drove me over to the student infirmary. I got the head doctor at the infirmary to see me. I told him what I had done and whimpered and pleaded for a diet. He looked up through his bushy eyebrows and (I'll never forget his words) said: "Don't eat so much." Brilliant. As soon as he said that, I got hungry again.

Of course, he was the last doctor I saw for several years. Back to the vicious cycle. There was absolutely no way on God's green earth that I could cheat on a diet and then go back on that diet. It didn't work. Every diet I found operated like a crash diet. I was always bailing out.

The reason is simple. I didn't know what I was doing. There was no plan I could follow. I didn't have control. I wasn't organizing my body to diet by feeding it what it needed while denying it what it didn't.

Finally, I figured out Controlled Cheating for myself. Cheating has been with us since dieting began, when Cindy and Clyde Cavepersons couldn't fit into their dinosaur-skin bikinis. Since cheating couldn't be avoided or abolished, there had to be a way to make it fit into my scheme of things, to make it work for, not against, the diet.

Out of desperation and need, I analyzed how I ate and subsequently how other fatties ate. No true eater can stop with one slice of cinnamon toast. It's not normal. Overweight people don't eat like other folks. If they did, they wouldn't be fat. I can't count the number of dates I've had who have said, after eating three French fries, "I'm stuffed." Of course, she weighed 102 pounds and complained about how fat she was.

As any good burglar knows, a lock must release to work smoothly. The dieting key is the desire and need to go back on the diet. The key and the release of Controlled Cheating work smoothly together because you have your Controlled Cheating Days to provide an outlet for that all-important key.

Everyone who diets is going to cheat. As sure as there isn't enough chocolate in the world, people on diets are going to cheat. Then after they cheat, the guilt, bad feelings, and food depression sets in. Every other fatty will scream at the heavens, "What's the use! I just can't do it. I'm weak and nothing but a fat slob."

To go on a diet that never gives you the opportunity to cheat is not realistic. Not only that, it's a pie in the face of what overweight human beings actually do. It's an insult to us.

The main reason why people can't lose weight and keep it off is that they can't go back on their diet once they cheat. Controlled Cheating totally eliminates that problem. You and I have our Controlled Cheating Days and cheating is built into our lives. No guilt, no depression afterward. We need it, we deserve it, and, with Fats Goldberg, we get it!

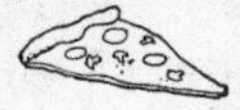

Hooray, Hurrah, Congratulations, You Get Another Controlled Cheatin' Day

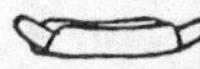

"Good afternoon, everybody. This is Howard Cashew from the House That Baby Ruth Built.

"You, the Controlled Cheater have just hit a stand-up triple over Joe DiMacaroni's head in deep center field.

"Because you're such a powerful, Controlled hitter, you're three-fourths of the way home to your Goal Weight. Now you get an extra Controlled Cheating Day.

"Congratulations. I give you a banana B.B. Bat taffy sucker."

Knowing you, you've already thumbed through this book and seen that your swiftly slimming silhouette can afford another Controlled Cheating Day.

Yes! Your mind and body can now handle an extra goody day because you've got your Controlled Cheating batting swing in a great low-cal groove.

Good ol' dieting, like good ol' baseball, has become the national pastime. But losing weight and keeping it off is more toil than a pleasant afternoon in the Wrigley Field bleachers getting a beautiful tan, an icy beer in one hand, a juicy hot dog with plenty of yellow mustard in the other, and two bags of peanuts roasting in your lap. By now you know it's a full-time job. Every day, not only must you get up and either put on makeup or scrape those tough whiskers off your face, you must also go right to work on your Controlled Cheating.

Look at it this way. You're the head honcho, boss, supervisor, foreman, union, and only employee. We Controlled Cheaters take our orders from a whole raft of barking bosses all screaming from inside our own beautiful skins. Cheating Eating is no eight-hour-a-day job, either. It's twenty-four hours a day, seven days a week—and no doughnut and coffee breaks (except on those you-know-when days).

You've already got one day off and now because you've been such a loyal and hard worker you can take another day off. Hooray! You also get a two-week eating vacation, which we'll talk about in a later chapter, and you didn't even have to go on strike. That's some good job.

Don't go nuts from all the excitement. There's no retirement from the job. No gold watch. No little house on the coast of Florida where you can grow your own sugarcane and watch the sun set over the top of your Lorna Doones.

What you do get is a life of good health and thinness. Controlled Cheating is the best job in the world. You're in business for yourself. And *yourself* is the business. All the decisions and rewards are yours. Controlled Cheating is a good time. And who wants to retire from a good time, anyway?

Controlled Cheating didn't come down from the sky all of a sudden more than two fast decades ago on a butter-flavored golden beam to bathe me in its spectacular light. I had no idea what I was doing. I *did know* that what I had been doing the first twenty-five years of my life sure wasn't working. I knew I had to cheat. That was a fat fact of life—my life.

I also knew that what I was doing *was* working. I didn't call it Controlled Cheating until 1961 or 1962. Before that, I didn't call it controlled or even cheating. I called it "I get to eat on Mondays."

What I did decide was that it was better to cheat on one day rather than all seven. That it was better to live with one day of eating what I wanted to, with good sense, rather than no days of fun food. That I could finally lose weight and keep it off on my program. That it was better to control and plan what I was doing rather than shooting up and down all the time like an express elevator in the Empire State Building.

During the first year of my diet, from 1959 to 1960, when I dropped from over 325 to 190, I thought the only time God was going to let me have to eat my precious goodies was one lonely day a week. The thought never flashed through my curly head that someday I would be able to cheat twice a week and, wow, finally every third day. One day a week was okay. I was almost normal weight, 175 pounds, happy, in good health, and had enough energy to rassle with a grizzly.

All of a sudden in 1968, I was in the Goldberg's Pizzeria business, standing in front of two 650-degree roaring ovens for ten hours a day schlepping pizzas. Boy, that needle on the old Health-O-Meter whizzed down like my body was in a severe economic recession. One sunny Sunday morning the scale shouted 160. Joyfully, prancing off the scale, the spectacular thought hit me that maybe, just maybe, I could cheat *twice* a week.

At first, I told myself, "Nah, you can't do that, Goldberg. You've been slim for ten years and all of a sudden you want to fool around with success. You must be some kind of a dieting dummy. You're going to be off and eating like the old days. Why blow ten years of the good thin life?"

But I couldn't stop it. The glorious thought of two Cheating Days kept whizzing through my brain. Naturally, my being a fat man only disguised as a thin man, what else would I think about?

I stuck one hand in the mozzarella cheese and the other in the pepperoni. This was how I did my best meditating. I made the decision.

Mumbling to myself, which frightened two customers enough for them to bolt out the door dragging their half-eaten mushroom pizza with them, I said, "Look, big boy, you've done a great job the last eleven years. The chances of you going out of control are 'slim.' If it doesn't work, you haven't lost a thing. You can always go back to one Cheating Day a week. Big deal. Give it a shot."

In those days, I closed the pizza store on Mondays. Of course, I cheated on Mondays. I also took Thursday nights off. Thursdays would be the natural time to add the Cheating Day. I could have another hot date and there were three days to lose the weight I would gain between Thursday and Monday.

I tried it and I liked it. My body and mind said thanks, too. I didn't shoot up and start gaining again as I feared. *I even lost another 10 pounds.*

With either two or three days between Controlled Cheating Days, I found I easily lost the weight I added on those days. I became smarter in my cheating, lived a more normal life, and I learned to "Double My Pleasure and Double My Fun."

But I was still rigid about my Cheating Days; only Mondays and Thursdays, for five more years. When I started franchising my pizza places, I had Saturdays and Sundays off. Saturday would be a great day to cheat. I could have a Saturday night date (if I could find one). There were more rip-roaring social events on Saturdays and I could have half a weekend for some giggles.

Fear, again, reared its ugly tummy. I was afraid to change those days from Monday and Thursday to Wednesday and Saturday. Still, after fifteen solid years of Controlled Cheating, I was quaking in my size 11D boots, afraid I was going to blow my thinness. You've probably already got the crystal-clear message that it takes me a long time to change. At least when it comes to Controlled Cheating.

Sticking one hand in the pizza dough and the other in the anchovies (I changed my meditating spots, too), I said, "Full mouth ahead." Changing the Cheating Days worked out fine.

So in twenty years of Controlled Cheating Eating, I have changed my program only three times. Deep down, this was fine with me; when it comes to losing weight and keeping it off, slow and steady is best. The last change came in 1979, when I started Controlled Cheating every third day. But like one of those Saturday afternoon Hopalong Cassidy serials, you'll have to wait for more on this in a later episode.

RULES AND REGULATIONS FOR THE GREAT AMERICAN EATING GAME OF CONTROLLED CHEATING FOR PEOPLE THREE-FOURTHS OF THE WAY TO THEIR GOAL WEIGHT

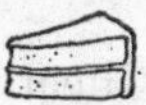

You're standing on third base, a little winded, where you've just earned another Cheating Day. The applause and screams are rolling out of the stands engulfing your thinning figure. One adoring fan ran out to get your autograph. Being the "aw shucks" star that you are, you, of course, graciously scribbled your signature in Jarlsburg cheese.

Don't get too cocky and take a big lead off third base and try a suicide steal of home plate. You've made it to third base and three-fourths of the way home to your Goal Weight through hard work and determination. You're on my team and I'm still the manager, Billy Sundae. You wait for the right signals. There are only a few rules and regulations you must stick to, but they are vitally important to your game plan.

YOUR EXTRA CONTROLLED CHEATING DAY MUST BE TWO OR THREE DAYS APART. THEY ARE *NOT* TO BE TWO DAYS IN A ROW

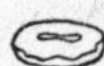

Most folks are off on Saturday and Sunday. I know what you're thinking: Those days sure would be ideal to cheat. Back off now. Two days in a row are dangerous even if they're Wednesday and Thursday.

1. Two straight Cheating Eating Days will give you too big a weight gain, not to mention a third-degree case of heartburn. This will make you twitchy, depressed, and frustrated.

You might get so nervous you'd blow the whole program and sprint toward Uncontrolled Cheating. Fat City, here you come again.

At this point in Controlled Cheating, too many cheeseburgers with grilled onions is too big a load for your slimming mind and body. There would be too many lines on the scale that would have to be lost.

2. Splitting the two days will let your body and mind lose the pounds you've gained so easily. Plus, you'll lose more weight as you roll to your Goal Weight.

Your Goal Weight is still on the beautiful horizon and you must keep on trekking. I don't want any detours to roadside refreshment stands.

3. Now that you're Cheating Eating two days, your weight loss will slow down. This is fine and dandy. You don't have that far to go now and you should slow down and smell the flours.

Everything is under control. You're dieting and Control Cheating correctly. There's no reason to get upset if you don't lose the rest of the weight in nineteen minutes. You didn't put it on in nineteen minutes. (Knowing you, though, maybe you did—like me!)

4. When you break up the days, you can mess up one Cheating Day and you still have another big day a couple of steps down the road.

"Messing up" means eating stupid, empty, high-calorie foods you didn't genuinely crave. You ate them because it was a Cheating Day and you had a couple of empty hands.

I've done this about 2,000 times in my Cheating Eating life. There I am, on my day, no diet, no date, no social event, just standing in the middle of Second Avenue with nothing to do but eat. And I run around eating ridiculous stuff only because I can do it that day. I pile on foods that don't get me truly excited.

For instance, gallons of high-calorie soda that gives me no food fix but dulls the appetite with empty calories. Then I move on to those terrible gummy little supermarket cakes, maybe a cold hot dog on a bun that was baked for the soldiers in the War of 1812. Or I drop in a grease pit where I know the food would turn off a trash compactor.

I don't have to be alone either. It could be at someone's house for a lousy dinner or I'd go out with pals and get bad eats plus spending a Brink's truck full of money. A double whammy. A wasted day. But it's isolated. No next day to compound the damage. Instead, immediate retraction. And a wait till the next Cheating Day for the guilt to recede.

The feeling I want you to have as you tuck yourself in at the end of a Cheating Day is one of a pleasant glow of eating satisfaction. Before you close your eyes, you drift back over the day and smile that there wasn't one wasted calorie.

The next morning you'll hop on the scale and grin because those couple of pounds you gained would be worth it. You go back to your low-calorie balanced diet with no regrets and a quick takeoff and additional loss.

5. With the Cheating Days split up, you always have something great to look forward to. Instead of one distant light of eating at the end of a long, low-calorie tunnel, you have two bright lights in two short blocks. You'll feel good.

BOZO EATING

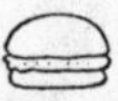

Did you ever see the movie *King Solomon's Mines?* It's undoubtedly the best adventure flick of all time. And every great adventure has secrets, mysteries, and surprises. I've probably seen it ten or fifteen times. If it ever comes your way, don't miss it. In fact, give me a call and we'll go together. You bring a yard and a half of hot buttered popcorn and I'll bring a six-pack of Pepsi with a lot of ice. Of course, we have to go on a Cheating Day.

The only thing I'm going to tell you about the movie is that Stewart Granger is this great hunter. Then there's beautiful Deborah Kerr, who sails to Africa from jolly old England to find her wayward husband who has vanished in darkest Africa while horsing around trying to dig up the fabulously rich Lost Mines of Solomon.

In *this* book, I fantasize that I'm a sort of no-shoulders Stewart Granger. Instead of being a great hunter, let's say I'm a small prospector. You and I are on this high adventure, looking for the thin body you camouflaged a long time ago under a protective coating of fat. I know this dangerous, uncharted territory because it took me twenty-five years to find my own thin self.

Here we are on this great escapade with loads of secrets, mysteries, surprises, and, of course, a happy ending for you.

I call it Bozo Eating.

SECRETS: BOZO EATING

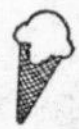

Bozo or nutsy or crazy eating is ramming, jamming, stuffing, sliding, and maneuvering all the delicious goodies you can get into your mouth at the same time. You do this whether you're hungry or not, and you go bozo only because it's a Cheating Day. Deep down you feel that you must get as much food as you can behind your cute little navel, because tomorrow is a Diet Day.

Ah, you've been a good, top-flight Controlled Cheater for a while now, and you have gotten this wonderful feeling that crazy, bozo hogging-it-up eating doesn't always satisfy you. Hold on: The truth is that eating only when you're hungry is much more satisfying and fun.

It only took me fifteen years to finally discover why my Controlled Cheating Days weren't quite doing the job. I discovered that if I waited until I was good and hungry, I had a more bozo time than when I ate solely because I could with no guilt or restrictions.

In my early Cheating Eating Days, I used to start chewing even if I had nothing in my mouth. The teeth were going up and down and sideways and grinding, if I was only ¼ inch below that completely stuffed open-the-top-button feeling.

It makes no difference whether you want to eat a pretzel with yellow mustard or lobster tails with a quart of drawn butter.

When you genuinely want to eat and you're hungry, you are going to enjoy what you're eating 1,000 percent more than when you're so full the tacos are inching out of your ears.

Ah, sweet secrets of life and eating.

MYSTERY

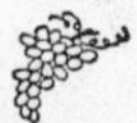

I love a mystery. Everyone gets all tingly when skeletons fall out of corn cob-webbed closets, gnarled bacon-greased hands come out from behind heavy, chocolate-brown velvet drapes and circle the beautiful neck of a screaming cook who forgot to put the fresh bread on the table when she laid out the chunky peanut butter and grape jelly.

One mystery that scares me and makes me laugh the most is when I discover something that I didn't know before about my skinny body.

Good mysteries take time to unfold with false clues, strange wild eyes peering out of creaky doors and evil-looking villains, who are prime suspects, but had nothing to do with the mystery.

A mystery that will always baffle me is that, when I started eating only when I got hungry on Controlled Cheating Days, several wonderful things happened:

1. My eating habits became more normal. I know that the way I eat will never become the way born skinnies eat. However, it's a heck of an improvement over the way I used to do it.

2. I actually ate less.

3. I had a better time and more fun than when I was hoisting in the goodies like a steam shovel.

The mystery is that a former fatty like me, who lives to eat, who would kill for a cashew, and who on a Diet Day has a constant edge of being hungry, *can* eat only foods that I truly ache for and have a giggling Cheating Day better than one on which I would eat like an unclogged drain in my kitchen sink.

Sure the body must change. I don't know how or why. I haven't lost the constant urge to eat, but I have become rational in my eating. Hooray for big favors.

Your body will change, too. With Controlled Cheating you will listen more to your body and feel what it wants and doesn't want. You'll also feel terrific mentally and physically that you have a natural control over your eating.

"Ah, sugar-sweet mystery of life."

SURPRISE

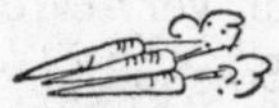

You'll become more relaxed about your eating on both your Diet Days and Cheating Eating Days.

With two days, there isn't the constant pressure of sprinting out of the house, munching on the dandelions sprouting between the cracks in the sidewalk, until you can get to your local doughnut store.

Waking up, you'll take a long, luxurious, relaxing stretch and realize that you have a terrific Controlled Cheating Day ahead of you. Don't get frightened. Cheating Days will never become a bore. There will always be that air of excitement and electricity. Folks on the bus will stare because your head will gleam like a 250-watt bulb. But you'll have a relaxed glow.

The basic you will not change when it comes to eating. For us former fatties, eternal vigilance is and must be our constant companion. Becoming more relaxed will make you stronger because now you know that you can lose weight and keep it off permanently.

Surprise: You never thought it could happen.

A LITTLE FLEXIBILITY, PLEASE

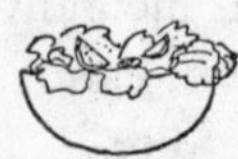

Now that you've reached two fabulous Cheating Days a week, you're a tough enough low-cal cookie to have a little flexibility.

Remember. Always and always. Forever and ever. You CANNOT have two Controlled Cheating Days in a row. Consecutive is a four-letter word. You can very carefully *switch* days though. Aren't I simply marvelous? So good to you!

Suppose you originally chose Sunday and Thursday and now you want to change the days to Wednesday and Saturday. You *cannot* cheat on Thursday and again on Saturday. You can, dear dieter, cheat on Sunday and then cheat again on Wednesday to start your new Cheating Day schedule. Or Tuesday and Saturday. Or whatever.

Plus you must be very, very careful when it comes to switching. Don't give yourself four Cheating Days in the transition week and think that neither your scale nor I will know the difference. We will.

After all the tummy-to-tummy conversations we've had, you know as well as I do the reasons for my, and your, being this tough. But let's go over it again for those of you in the second balcony who couldn't hear all the lines.

1. Having less than two days between Cheating Eating Days doesn't give your body enough time to lose the weight you've gained. Which is lethal for you physically and mentally.

2. If you continually mess around with your days, pretty quick you'll lose the set routine and guess what? Big Person's Shops, here you come again.

Flexibility doesn't mean anything goes. It says that now you can use your free will, sort of.

YOU MUST GO BACK ON YOUR DIET!

As you're licking your finger, to turn the page to the next chapter, guess what's coming? You're right!

YOU MUST GO BACK ON YOUR DIET!

YOU
MUST
GO
BACK
ON
YOUR
DIET,
BABY!

AFTER ANY CHEATING DAY.

Being able to Control Cheat 50 percent of the time is easier than Cheating Every Third Day.

Sadly, I must tell you this system doesn't work. Our bodies cannot adjust and lose the weight we've put on in only one day of dieting. I tried. Boy, did I try—twice. I found myself sliding toward cheating every day. You know what that means. "Kiss Today Good-bye."

Every word in this book has been kitchen-tested for you, kitchen-tested in the best laboratory I know, my lean, bony body. Trust me and don't try it. Every-other-day cheating emphatically doesn't work. Be content and happy with Controlled Cheating Every Third Day. It's what you deserve.

HOW I DISCOVERED EVERY-THIRD-DAY CHEATING AND GAINED HAPPINESS BUT NOT WEIGHT

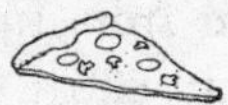

In October 1978, as TWA Flight 86 came in for a landing at LaGuardia Airport, the Boeing 727 was tilting slightly to the right. And it wasn't because Ronald Reagan might have been on board either. Fats Goldberg was coming back from his twice yearly eating trip to Kansas City, where he gained the usual seventeen pounds in seven days.

Going back to my two-and-a-half-room apartment, I unpacked my Arthur Bryant's barbecued ribs and cinnamon twists from Lamar's Donuts. I sat down dejected. This was the last eating day of my twice yearly Cheating Vacation. I had nothing to look forward to but six straight days of cold-turkey dieting until I could cheat again.

I didn't mind the six days of low-calorie, balanced dieting. This had been an old routine of mine for twenty years. What bothered me was that I was looking at only two Cheating Days a week for another six months.

Two Cheating Days felt like nothing when I had just had seven consecutive championship eating days. Life wasn't fair. There had to be a better way. But I knew if I could find my way out of the airport, I could find a way out of this dilemma.

I felt low down and twitchy. I looked at the encrusted carmel corn under my fingernails. Here I was forty-five years old. How much time did I have left? I wanted to live as long as I possibly could, and eating was so much fun. As I stared down at my Nike running shoes, the laces became soaked with my tears and everything became a blur. From the haze, a thought arose. Why not cheat every third day?

I got so excited I jumped straight up in my old Yankee Stadium seat. The New York State Lottery at that instant posted the odds at ninety-nine to one that I could handle the extra Cheating Days.

I whipped out my calendar from the Gaiety Delicatessen and counted the total days I could cheat, if I Cheated Every Third Day.

Using all my fingers and toes, I calculated that I'd be able to cheat 121 days in 1979. Comparing that with 104 days of Controlled Cheating twice a week gave me seventeen more days of happiness. Every year!

"Hold on, Fatberg," I said to myself. "Is this another one of the cons and tricks you like to play on yourself so you can sneak in more eating? Remember what happened when you tried cheating every other day? You gave it a fling not once, but twice, and you almost threw yourself into your old 320-pound orbit."

Then I said, "Hush up. What can it hurt if I find that I didn't lose the weight I put on after a Cheating Day in two days. I can always diet the extra day, which I have been doing anyway for the last eleven years. There isn't any risk." The odds went off the board because I knew I could do it successfully.

Eating Every Third Day worked great. My body liked it and so did my pals. Now, because of the flexibility, when I was invited to a big gathering, I could go and eat something besides carrot sticks and limp celery. Before I'd have to whine, "Oh, I sure would like to come, but I can't eat."

Every Third Day Eating gives you almost everything except Uncontrolled Cheating. It normalizes your Cheating Eating habits even more than the twice-a-week eating plan. It makes your eating life as fun and flexible as a strand of freshly cooked spaghetti hanging off your chin. Plus, with 121 days of Controlled Cheating out of 365 each year, you have ONE-THIRD of your life in which to eat good!

This was only the third change in twenty-one years I've made in my Controlled Cheating Program and I'm totally convinced this is the final modification to make on the Gravy Train.

BOZO EATING

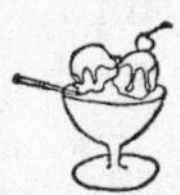

Your next guest on HHHHHHHEEEEEERRRRRREE'S YOU has been a visitor on the show before. Here's the Clown of Cheating, Bozo "Crazy" Eating. Let's give Bozo a big boo.

This is the last time "Crazy" will be a guest. I invited him back once more so you can see that she or he is not very funny, tells "tasteless" jokes, and doesn't have much to say except, "Give me more to eat." So let's get this rude person on and off in a hurry.

You're at Goal Weight now and a professional Controlled Cheater. Being a whiz at controlling your weight, you know that Uncontrollable Cheating on your Cheating Days doesn't work.

1. Stuffing it in, just because you can, doesn't satisfy your basic cheating need to eat. That is the need to emphatically cheat with foods *you want*. The really good times roll (and butter) on your Cheating Days when you're hungry enough to eat a Mack Truck, tires and all. And you get to eat foods you truly crave with no guilt or twitch because it's planned.

2. Your favorite foods taste even more sensational when you lust hungrily after them, like a big slice of strawberry cheesecake when you're hungry. Eating that cheesecake when you're full is useless and dumb. That fork is moving senselessly from the plate to your mouth and back again like a carnival Ferris wheel, around and around, but with no squeals of delight.

You're not getting the full flavor and sensory excitement that delicious creamy cheesecake with the sugary fresh strawberries can give you. This is why planning is so important on your Controlled Cheating Day.

3. Dancing on the scale the morning after your Controlled Cheating Day and the needle stops two or three notches above your Goal Weight, I want you to delightfully dream back over yesterday. Yes, and know that you ate almost everything you wanted and got the full enjoyment from the day, not that you slapped on needless pounds without your tongue smiling.

4. One of the great pleasures of Cheating Eating is on your Diet Days when the hunger gets tough and you can fantasize and daydream about what you're going to eat on your next Cheating Day, which is only two days away. Make every bite count, even in your dreams.

YOUR BODY CHANGES

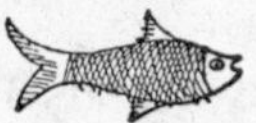

How do you like your new body? Looks good. You fit into jeans you haven't been able to button in six years. You've not only lost pounds but inches, too. The little economy car you bought finally fits without giving you a ridge in your stomach from the steering wheel. Your shoes are even flopping around your feet. You didn't know you could lose weight in your toes, did you?

Friends keep yelling, "Boy, do you look terrific. How much did you lose? Wish I could lose weight."

You're now a certifiable skinny. That's the outside of your body, the part everyone can see and which gives you such great pleasure. Bask in the glory; you deserve it.

A new you has emerged from your heavy overcoat of fat. By now you know that losing weight and keeping it off starts from the inside and works its way out.

You start by doing. Dieting is doing; it is an active verb. Don't start by trying to analyze everything you do before, during, and after you eat. If you do, you'll waste all your time trying to go deep into the recesses of your mind while your hand is going deeper into the bag of nacho-flavored Doritos.

Self-analysis is important and this comes as you're dieting, losing weight, and keeping it off. Every day that you're alive, new ideas, insights, and revelations will come to you naturally. Folks who keep analyzing without doing anything are copping out. They're waiting for that great beam from the sky to take them away to a skinny never-never land. In losing weight and keeping it off, YOU LEARN BY DOING.

Right now you're at the weight you want to be. You've probably learned more about yourself during this Controlled Cheating Period than ever before.

Maybe now you can understand why you got fat in the first place, why you kept eating, and how you're going to stay at your Goal Weight.

Every day of the twenty-two years I've been Cheating Eating I've learned something new about myself. Sometimes it comes in little bits and pieces until I get the whole idea.

I'm writing this on a Sunday, a Cheating Day. I just came back from brunch where I had a combination corned beef and salami omelet, French fries, a toasted buttered bagel, and two cups of coffee. Tonight I have a date. What I want for dinner is real food, not empty calories, but Italian, Mexican, or Chinese food.

(I'm writing this the next day, Monday. We chose Chinese: sweet and pungent shrimp, chicken lo mein, pineapple chunks, and fortune cookies. My date has a tiny appetite, so I ate most of hers, too. On the way back to her apartment, I had a rum raisin ice cream cone.)

Over the last several years my tastes have changed. My craving for food is still the same and I'm still as hungry as before, but my desire for sugary foods has gone down. I suspect I've developed more sophisticated tastes, that want a variety of foods, not just the same old jelly-roll stand-bys of my youth. Ten years ago, I would have given you a lifetime of pizzas if you'd have told me that was going to happen. Oh sure, I still love ice cream, cakes, pies, and anything else with a sweet taste, but what I want even more on my Controlled Cheating Days are things like pasta, all different kinds of bread and butter, cheeses, fried chicken, steak, and chili. And all sorts of new, never-before-experienced restaurants: Argentinian, Czechoslovakian, Spanish, and Japanese. I want to experiment and enjoy it all.

Where you are now, a Controlled Cheater who has reached Goal Weight, is a wonderful coordination of mind and body that has proven that you can do most anything you want in life.

What's left of you deserves a big hug.

DIET DON'TS

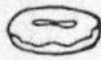

You're the real thing, the genuine article. You've reached your Goal Weight and you're worthy of a mountain of congratulatory telegrams, ovations, cheers, and tributes. (And raviolis.)

Beware, Goal Weighter, of Diet Don'ts. I must warn you about these. They are obnoxious habits that will plunge your popularity to about the level of a vacation weekend at a Siberian work camp.

Time to confess. I used to be guilty of all these offenses. Maybe if you check yourself before you begin, it might save you many Saturday nights home alone.

The Diet Snob

A former fatty who swaggers down the street with an air of superiority looking down at folks who are overweight. Diet Snobs say to themselves, "Look at those fat slobs who can't control themselves. See that one at the soda fountain with the root beer float and the slice of chocolate cream pie. He's not as self-disciplined or as wonderfully thin as I am." A Diet Snob scolds, huffs, and puffs about other people who can't control themselves. Remember, Goal Weighter, you're always one step away from Fat City yourself.

The Diet Bore

Former fatties who have lost weight and cannot stop talking about it. All their pals know every morsel they've eaten that day, what the scale said, what they're going to Cheat Eat with on their Controlled Cheating Days, and on which days they can cheat.

When asked how they did it, they go on and on until two people get ill or someone finally says, "I'm sorry I asked." Plus every dinner conversation is sprinkled with long lists of what they can and cannot eat.

Diet Bores always talk in a loud enough voice to take blue ribbons at an Ozark Hog-Calling Contest. Well, it takes one to know one, as they say. And hogging conversation with your diet talk is as unappetizing as hogging food (the way you did—but you don't do anymore).

Diet Martyr

A hot stuff dieter on a Non-Cheating Day who sits down to eat with someone else, their family, or at a banquet, who sadly and silently suffers with eyes cast down at the broiled fish and salad with fresh lemon dressing. The weight of the eating world is on their back and their chin is resting on the table. Oh pity me!

Diet Watcher

A tasteless Goal Weighter who stares at other people's food while they are eating. Each bite, taste, slurp, and crumb is recorded on the eyeballs lovingly and longingly by the Diet Watcher. This is the most dangerous of all Diet Don'ts. You could end up with a plate of hot lasagne in the face.

Take heed of these little tips. Years ago I saw the eyes of friends glaze over with boredom and anger with my self-righteous nincompoopery. I'm lucky to have a chubby pal left.

YOU ARE RELAXED

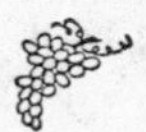

Have you got a big bargain in this book. For the measly $11.95, besides telling you how to lose weight and keep it off, I'm going to give you, at no extra charge, a selection of low-calorie mantras. These magic words are the keys to relaxing while at your Goal Weight, and while keeping your weight off on Diet Days, by having fun and talking to yourself.

A mantra is a word or phrase used in meditation, repeated over and over with eyes closed in a relaxed position until the mantra sinks into your subconscious and you become as limp as an old leaf of lettuce.

Most meditation techniques come from the East, mainly from India, where the meditation teachers of the future must study for years to learn how to teach the proper techniques for using the mantra. These Controlled Cheating mantras were taught to me by Swami Grease, who never got farther east than East St. Louis, Illinois.

Swami Grease received them in a solemn and beautiful ceremony from a candy vending machine man named Roy. This great teacher was refilling the candy machine with Snickers, Paydays, Butterfingers, and Reese's Peanut Butter Cups at the bus station in East St. Louis. Standing on his tiptoes between the vending machine and the trash barrel filled with sticky candy wrappers and empty Coke bottles, Swami Grease was whispered these secret mantras.

However, these powerful low-calorie mantras are used differently than the Eastern mantras I described earlier. You must never repeat my mantras with your eyes closed or in a relaxed position. They must be repeated only at times when you want to eat on a Diet Day, in front of an open empty refrigerator.

LOW-CALORIE MANTRAS

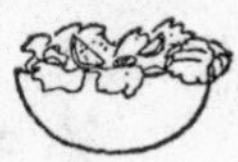

1. Will Power—Phooey; Will Power—Phooey
2. Goldberg Action; Goldberg Action
3. Smile; Smile
4. Relax and Take It Easy; Relax and Take It Easy
5. Prayer Can Work; Prayer Can Work
6. Low-Calorie, Balanced Diet; Low-Calorie, Balanced Diet
7. Exercise; Exercise
8. Controlled Cheating; Controlled Cheating
9. Goal Weight; Goal Weight

A
N
D

10. The Most Important Mantra of Them All

YOU MUST GO BACK ON YOUR DIET AFTER A CHEATING DAY

YOU MUST STAY ON YOUR DIET TWO DAYS AFTER A CHEATING DAY

YOU MUST NOT MAKE YOUR DIET A "DIATRIBE" FOR OTHERS

Weighty Matters

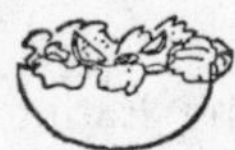

COME BACK, LITTLE CHEATER

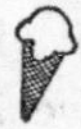

A Special Message from Your Old Pal Fats Goldberg

You tried this diet for six days and you were wonderful with low-calorie balanced dieting. Then came your first Controlled Cheating Day. You loved it so much you never went back to the diet part. Now it's six months later and you can't understand why you haven't lost a pound.

Or one month, six months, one year, or six years from now the same thing happens. You hit a Controlled Cheating Day and you can't stop. You are on that diet roller coaster again going straight up.

Although Controlled Cheating works well for most people, sometimes you can't help yourself and you fall off the Welcome Wagon. You can start again. We accept repeater cheaters, fallen angels, and other sugar-coated sinners. It's very easy to climb back on board in one simple step: JUST GO BACK TO PAGE ONE AND START ALL OVER AGAIN! I still like you.

DON'T GIVE UP YOUR DAY JOB

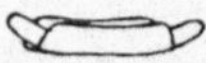

Cheating Eating Vacations didn't flash through my brain until after the first year I was on the diet and weighed a paltry 190.

I went back to Kansas City twice for vacations on the way down from 325 to 190, but I didn't cheat. Not cheating almost blew the whole program. I was walking around my personal eating wonderland where I'd put on the old original 325 and was not able to do anything except drive by the drive-ins.

I did take my regular once-a-week Controlled Cheating Day, but what's one day a week compared to seven days a week for twenty-five years? One day a week was all I thought I was ever going to get, even on vacations.

It was a good year, 1961. I was schlepping along in Chicago dieting and fairly happy. The dieting was tough as the bark on a tree, or easy as pie, or somewhere in between, depending on what day it was.

Over a long period of time, a revolutionary idea started in my toes and worked its way up to my Pepsi-soaked brain. *DIETING IS LIKE A JOB. A FULL-TIME JOB. YOUR SECOND JOB.* The more I thought about it the truer it became. Losing weight and keeping it off is *exactly* like a job. Each morning I had to get up and go to not one, but two, jobs.

One job was to slip on a Brooks Brothers suit, oxford-cloth shirt, rep tie, over-the-calf socks, and Florscheim Imperial plain-toed cordovans and go to work at the Chicago *Tribune*. The other was getting up every morning and going to my job of dieting. With dieting, I didn't have to go very far. Both were equally important. One was to give me enough loot to put bread on the table. The other job was not to eat it (except on Controlled Cheating Days).

You don't give up your regular job when you take on the additional task of dieting. You work at both. Don't worry. Moonlight becomes you, especially as you get slimmer and slimmer!

Losing weight and keeping it off is awakening each day to the job of taking care of your body. It's the same as getting up and taking care of the house and children, or going to the plant, office, store, truck, or construction site.

The Controlled Cheating Program I was doing successfully was a full-time job, the same as my other business but with some big differences.

1. Keeping slim is a twenty-four-hour-a-day duty, not an eight-hour deal with time and a half for overtime. We don't get paid with more food for working overtime on a diet.

2. There are no foremen, bosses, or other honchos to keep an eye on what you're doing and telling and showing you what to do. *You're totally in business for yourself!*

When I noodled out that Controlled Cheating was a job, I also figured this was one of the main reasons why I, like most other fatties, couldn't lose weight and keep it off. We were looking at the problem in the wrong way.

All the time we'd think we could go on a diet for a while, maybe lose all the weight we wanted and then relax and never put it on again. That's dead wrong.

At our jobs where we get paid, we don't work hard for a while and then relax and expect to get paid for the rest of our lives. If we did that, we wouldn't have the job. Why should dieting be any different? We have to get up every morning and GO TO DIETING, like any job. Holding down two jobs is mean stuff. It takes hard work and everything we've got.

Hold on. Since dieting is like some tough job, how 'bout we get some of the benefits and goodies straight jobs have? We do. We do.

With Controlled Cheating in 1961, I had a day off, like my money job. As you know by now, we have every third day off, which is actually better than your regular job.

Again in 1961, I said, what about a two-week vacation? Why not try? When I did go to Kansas City on vacation, and had to diet, I was miserable. I thought, let me cheat for seven straight days and see if I can shake those pounds off when I get back.

In the spring of 1962, I drove to Kansas City in my 1956 Chevy. Laughing all the way down Route 66, Highways 36, 54, and 40, I ate and vacationed for a week. In seven days, I put on fifteen pounds. It was staggering, but boy, did I have a super-sensational vacation.

Sure, when I came back, I had to start dieting again. Who cared? With seven days of eating behind me, I could come back and go on my diet again, and I knew I was home free when it came to staying skinny the rest of my life.

Two months later I had lost the fifteen pounds. You've got to remember that I started my Controlled Cheating again immediately as you will too after six days of dieting.

That was nineteen years ago and I still vacation and eat seven straight days twice a year. This job works and will work for you, too.

Some final points:

1. You can never retire from your diet job as you can from your straight job. No gold watch, no Social Security, no good-bye party. There is no job security either. You can never be secure when dieting. But you'll live a long and happy life.

2. You'll never get a raise, especially in pounds. Thank God!

ODE TO MY HEALTH-O-METER

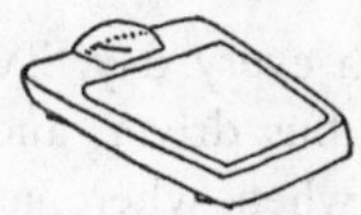

When I die at the age of ninety-three, I want my faithful and trusty Health-O-Meter scale for my tombstone. If the cemetery won't allow ancient scales for headstones, then I'm going to have it buried with me in my plain pine box. They say you can't take it with you, but I'm going to prove them wrong. (Who are "they" anyway?)

No one knows what's on the other side. Maybe, just maybe, there will be a "Fat Heaven" where we can eat all we want and never get fat. What a "heaven" it would be, with cherry and apple pies growing on trees and fettucini Alfredo sprouting from the ground. If this happens, then I'll still give my scale a proper place of honor, next to my hanging Pepsi plant.

Suppose, on the other hand, I have to diet for eternity. Then I'll surely need my scale. Anyway I look at it, there is no way I'm leaving without it.

One reason I'm not married is that I'm deeply in love with my scale. It's a real love/hate relationship, though. That sweetheart on the bathroom floor never lies. I've talked to it, cussed it, and caressed it. The scale's my friend on thin days and I hate it on fat days, depending on where that big black needle stops.

The year when I went from 325 to 190, I weighed myself when I got up, after I went to the bathroom, before I got dressed, when I came home from work, before I ate, after I ate, and before I went to bed. On weekends, sometimes in the middle of the afternoon I'd strip down and weigh to see how things were going.

For the last twenty-one years, I've managed to restrain myself to once a day in the morning without my clothes. This takes all my Goldberg Action, but I think I've got that craziness licked.

Weighing Every Day

You and I should weigh every day. Everyone in the diet, nutrition, medical, waitress, bus driver, and every other field, has their own pet theories on when, where, and how to weigh. Their guesses range all the way from three times a day to once a month. I've never seen anything about once a year. Probably because the people who tell you to do it can't see the scale over their stomachs.

I have my own time- and pain-tested reasons why I hop on the scale every morning. I weigh every day because I like good news. I want my morale boosted. I want to see how I'm doing as soon as possible. Eternal vigilance, again, is one of the keys to successful Controlled Cheating.

I don't want any surprises. Every three days, every week, or month is too long for me to wait. I want an immediate answer on how I'm doing.

Getting up every morning, I make my bed (whoever invented fitted sheets should get the Congressional Medal of Honor from the bachelors of America), shuffle sleepily into the bathroom without any clothes on and, after elimination, get on the Health-O-Meter. Besides telling me how I did yesterday, this is a sure waker-upper. All I have to do is step on the scale and get a surprise down or up, and I wake up faster than if Loni Anderson came in, dragged me out of bed, and threw me on an iceberg.

About six or seven years ago, I decided to *try* weighing once a week. The original reason was to reduce my daily scale tension. This way I could really get nervous only once a week. Sure I could handle once a week on Saturday mornings, the morning of one of my Cheating Eating Days. I'd been a successful skinny for fifteen years. What could be bad? What could happen?

Here's what could happen. The first week was fine. I did my normal Controlled Cheating, hopped on the scale Saturday morning, and I was still at my original Goal Weight. This was easy and wonderful.

The second week I cheated on my two days. BUT on my low-calorie balanced diet days, I started horsing around a little bit: another half a bagel here, a cup of ice cream there. I said to myself, "Take it easy. You can take it off toward the end of the week and you can still come in under the wire at your original Goal Weight on Saturday morning."

Quit grinning! You guessed what happened. I danced on the scale Saturday morning and my farsighted eyes almost fell on the dial like marbles. I had slapped on four big ones over my Goal Weight.

I looked to see if anyone was standing on the scale with me. My palms became rivers of nervous perspiration. A deep rumble started in my appendix; up through my quivering body and out of my tortured mouth came a scream of terror that would make the late Alfred Hitchcock's jowls shake.

That was it. No more weighing once a week. Everyday weighing was my one-way ticket to thinness.

Fluctuations and Plateaus

Our weight fluctuates, especially when we're losing. Don't get discouraged if the dial does the Mashed Potato. During the first weeks of dieting and Controlled Cheating, our bodies have to adjust to the new program.

There are physiological changes that arbitrarily happen that have nothing to do with how you're dieting and Control Cheating. You might be retaining some water or eating too much salt. As long as you're following your low-calorie, balanced diet program, you'll be fine.

You are going to see fluctuations. The scale is a teacher from whom you can learn something about your body. There's no way you're going to see a weight loss every day. You have to accept that losses will come slowly. But as long as they eventually do come, you're okay.

Everybody loses weight at different rates. Some folks drop a lot at the beginning. Some don't lose for a while and then it clicks. Not everyone loses at the same step. Everyone's stairs are different sizes. And some have landings. Some even have one long continuous staircase.

Sometimes I get real cocky and smart-alecky about my body. I think I can play my body like Erroll Garner can play the piano. No one watches what they eat and drink the way I do. If I eat certain diet foods, I'll lose so many pounds, I tell myself. Then I'm almost always shocked at how wrong I can be about forecasting my weight in the morning. So I stopped predicting. My body is a mystery. Everyone loves a mystery.

My body also plateaus. Now don't get jealous if your body doesn't plateau. That is, there are times I stay at the same weight regardless of what I eat or don't eat when dieting.

On the way down in 1959, there was a period when I got stuck at the same weight for about three weeks. I was eating the same amount of low-calorie foods, but the dumb needle wasn't moving. I was going crazy. I didn't know what to do. What was going on? I got discouraged. Maybe God wants me fat? No such luck. Finally I dropped five pounds in one day. Happily, I was off and running again.

When I had my annual physical exam in Chicago I asked Dr. Skom what happened. He said that my particular gorgeous, Adonis-type physique loses weight in stair steps. That is, I'll stay the same for a while and then take another step down. I told him I'd prefer sliding down the bannister.

Keep a close eye on your body and see how it operates. If it plateaus, relax and keep dieting. Eventually, you'll start skipping down those stairs again.

Magic with the Scale or Houdini with the Health-O-Meter

When it comes to con games and magic tricks with my scale, I make Paul Newman and Robert Redford in *The Sting* look like amateurs.

You've probably got your own magic tricks hidden up your sleeves that you use to make the scale read lighter. Alas, even for an old scale trickster like me, every magic act I try is only an *illusion*. We're not getting our real weight and we're kidding ourselves.

Heaven forbid that I corrupt you, but here are some of the old favorite hocus-pocus tricks I used to try pulling.

1. SLEIGHT OF HAND

Also called Slight of Hand. Picking up your scale and moving it to carpeting, which will make it register lighter than on a hard floor.

2. TIPPYTOE AND HEEL ROCK BAMBOOZLE

Standing on your toes to make the scale go down. Very hard on your toenails. Heel Rock is the opposite. You rock back on your heels, which could be dangerous due to the fact you may bounce into the bathtub. The problem with this trick is that it doesn't work.

3. MAKING THE SCALE DISAPPEAR

This works very well if you wear glasses and it's a simple illusion. Do not wear your glasses when you weigh. Squinting at the dial will automatically let you read a lower number. For those who don't wear glasses, think sad thoughts. Your eyes will tear and the scale will become a blur. Make up any weight you want.

4. THE SIDE BEND SNEAK

While standing on the scale, bend your body far to the right. When you look at the dial at this angle, the needle will be farther to the left where the numbers are smaller.

5. TOWEL BAR ILLUSION

As you are getting on the scale, grab hold of the towel bar with one hand, put the other in the sink, and press down. This way you can weigh anything you want. The Towel Bar Illusion can also be performed with an assistant. Have another person stand next to you while you're on the scale. With your forearm press down on the assistant's shoulder. You can also hold on to the wall or hang from the chandelier or shower curtain. If you use an assistant, make sure he or she has strong shoulders and is good-looking.

6. THE DISAPPEARING ACT

This works very well if you throw the scale out, smash it to bits, or leave it at someone's doorstep. You can always say the scale was too old and you have to buy a new one. This trick was taught to me by my friend Judy, a professional scale magician. In the last three years she has smashed five scales beyond recognition. Judy now has an iron and steel scale that is guaranteed indestructible. She recently retired from the profession.

7. TILE PLACEMENT FLIMFLAM

This is the oldest trick I have in my bag. The only problem is that it's never fooled anyone except me. I place the front end of the scale on the exact same tiles of my bathroom floor every morning. If I move the scale, I'm afraid the needle will soar. Heaven forbid if I ever moved from this apartment. I'd have to come back every morning to weigh myself.

All this trickery is top secret. Keep your magic scale illusions in your magic top hat along with your disappearing fat rabbit.

Do Not March to a Different Scale

In the good old days, when I was checking my weight every twenty-five minutes, I'd drop by daily at Marshall Field's on State Street in Chicago and weigh on every scale on the rack to see if I weighed less on any of them. Finally the sales folks got tired of seeing me and inquired politely whether I'd like to purchase one. I explained I had already bought one there and this was a form of hobby with me—trying out new scales.

One courteous saleslady explained that the hobby department was on another floor, but I could have visiting privileges once a week to see my old pals.

I also weighed in at friends' houses and apartments, strange doctors' offices, or anywhere there was something with a platform and numbers that would tell me how much I weighed.

Weighing on every scale you see is dangerous. Just because you see a scale at someone's house or in a department store or even in the meat department of your supermarket doesn't mean you have to climb on. You weigh differently at different times during the day. You also have clothes on. And all scales weigh differently.

I know what you're doing, you little devil, you. You're looking for a friendy gauge that will give you a lower number so you can feel better and maybe cheat a little bit more. But no way. This is the only way to weigh; to play the scale like a professional:

Please weigh every day in the morning, after elimination, on your own scale without your clothes on.

The Care and Feeding of the Scale

Or Taking Care of Your Friend on the Floor

You might think that once you buy a scale, you just take it home, throw it on the floor, and you can forget about it. You think you'll never touch your scale again, except with your feet, when you climb on board every morning. Pals, scales don't work that way. They have hearts and souls just like you. You take care of your dog, cat, crocodile, and Model-A Ford, so why should your scale be any different?

I caress, fondle, and talk to my scale like the friend it is. Once a week, I bathe my yellow-covered baby with Windex and wipe it dry with Bounty paper towels. I make doubly sure the plastic piece that covers the dial is crystal clear so I can get an accurate picture of my weight.

I keep my scale in the bathroom. But any place is fine. The kitchen is good because it could give you a warning before you whip open the refrigerator door.

If ever I redecorate my two and a half rooms, I'm going to center my luxurious new living room around my scale. I'll use it as a piece of free-form sculpture, right next to my Sony twelve-inch color TV, across from my battered rolltop desk with its Smith-Corona typewriter.

My scale and I will shortly announce our engagement. You'll be invited to the wedding. We'll be registered at Safeway. Don't worry about sizes or colors.

Buying a Scale

My scale is twenty-one years old. I've tried to buy a new scale many times. Every time I bring a new one home, I stare at it a couple of hours and end up taking it back. I just can't get myself to abandon my faithful friend. We've been through so much together.

This has been going on for many years now. Saturday afternoon is scale-shopping time. Other normal folks look for cheap underwear and catcher's mitts. I go through Bloomingdale's, Macy's, and every other store looking at the new fashions for weighing bodies.

I think I'm going to start a new business with a line of Goldberg's Designer Scales like all those designer jeans. I'll have a big flashy TV campaign with sexy women and men discoing up, down, and over The Scale with a big Goldberg's label on the rear.

I've bought at least seven new scales, but I've returned them all. I'm plain afraid of how they would read in the mornings. The new scale might hurt me. Back it goes.

If you are going to buy a new scale, make the investment in a good one. Don't get some cheap model that isn't absolutely accurate.

Most new scales have a little knob so that you can adjust the scale accurately. Once you've got your honest poundage, no fair messing with that dial again: *That's cheating.*

When I get rich my first big investment will be on a stand-up model, like my doctor has. I may never use it, but I'll enjoy looking at it. My status symbol.

ONE DAY AT A TIME

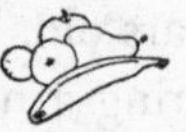

That's right. Do everything in this book one day at a time. TODAY is THE day. The only day in our lives. Yesterday is "Gone With The Wind" and you can't see tomorrow lurking around the corner, unless you have long eyeballs. We can do absolutely nothing about yesterday. Like that pound and a half of Hydrox Cookies you ate four years ago, it's all ancient history.

Regardless of what your horoscope predicts about meeting someone tall, dark, and rich, you can't tell what's going to happen. So why worry and stew about stuff that might or might not happen. No one has control over tomorrow.

On a Diet Day, zero in on eating a low-calorie, balanced diet for TODAY only. Why get twitchy about how many days you have to eat iceberg lettuce before you can cheat again? Diet for today ONLY!

When it's a Controlled Cheating Day, enjoy that glorious day to the fullest extent of the holes in your belt. Laugh, sing, dance, cavort, eat. Don't start thinking in the middle of the afternoon about tomorrow when you have to go back on your dumb diet.

Forget yesterday and tomorrow. Live for today. Today is the only twenty-four hours we've got for sure.

NAGGING

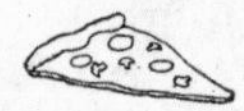

Just looking at that obscene word makes me angry. I've been nagged by experts most of my natural life. Nagging is the most negative thing you can do to an overweight person. Even looking at the way the letters fit together shows it's a truly foul word. Nagging gets my blood as hot as pizza cheese.

Fat people get nagged more than anyone else alive because their problem is right out there for everyone to see. We chubbies are large, hard-to-miss targets, so we're easy prey for every loudmouth. The earliest memories I have are of other kids teasing, kidding, and making fun of how fat I was. You know what they used to sing: "Fatty, fatty, two by four, couldn't get through the streetcar door."

The teasing went on until I could grab their skinny little bodies and sit on their legs. Eventually I developed a fast, mean mouth and could give back the kidding with even more knives attached. Shoot, I didn't win anything doing that either.

In all my experience, nagging, slamming, rapping, criticizing, or ragging has never gotten an overweight person to lose weight and keep it off. Nagging works exactly in the opposite way. What actually happens is that we fatties eat even more from anger and to show those gate mouths what we can really do.

Something I cannot understand about naggers (*we* are the naggees) is that they cannot get the idea through their stupid heads that WE KNOW we're fat. Naggers think they're giving us this brand-new piece of information hot off the wires. You bet we know we're fat. All it takes is a quick glance in the mirror to see our bulging clothes and a scalding case of heartburn—our constant reminders.

To their credit, naggers sincerely think and feel they are helping us. What they don't understand is that the way to really help us is to leave us alone, or else sit down with us and try to understand where we are in our Battle of the Bulge.

God bless my folks. They never nagged or criticized, although I knew they wanted to. Their leaving me alone was one of the main reasons why I eventually lost weight and kept it off. They let me figure it out for myself. They had confidence in me.

The only time I ever heard anything from my folks was occasionally when I was working in the market and I had my whole head, instead of just one hand, buried in a big box of Nabisco Vanilla Sandwich Cookies. They would just say, "Larry!" But this didn't stop me either.

Naggers come in all forms. They can be parents, brothers, sisters, friends, relatives, teachers, or someone who honestly does like you. Regardless, the results are always the same, a big ZERO.

Naggers feel they're superior to us. To their thin minds, all we need is a *little* push, a *little* yelling, a *little* nudge and we'll straighten out and become thin and perfect—just like them. If only it was that easy.

Naggers are always experts on other people's problems. Whether it's overeating, over or under anything. No wonder they call old beat-up, run-down, worthless horses NAGS. Why don't naggers nag themselves into faultless, flawless human beings? Who asked for their advice anyway? There are certain people I go to when I want advice. I trust their intelligence and judgment. I ask for it.

There's a great quote I remember when I get unwanted advice and guidance: "If you can tell good advice from bad advice, you don't need advice." (With free advice you get what you pay for.)

Now, the same people who nagged me when I was fat are still nagging, "You're much too thin. You could afford to put on a few pounds. We can see your bones!" I can never win, except with the folks that count with me.

People nagging at you won't help; you have to help yourself to dieting. But if the naggers are folks you otherwise like or have to live with, you'll just have to grit your teeth and put up with it . . . for a while. If the naggers won't stop, give it back to them with both barrels, with plenty of kidding and teasing about *their* weaknesses. Do it with a smile and make them laugh. The best defense is a good jolly offense.

The sole purpose of this book is to get you to re-examine your lives and eating habits and understand there is a way to lose weight and keep it off and still be a happy eater.

I promise I'll never nag you about it.

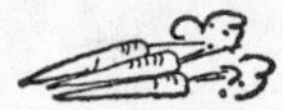

Exercise: Hiking and Biking with a Jewish Viking

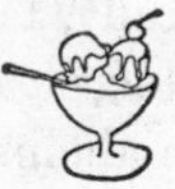

Your first and most important exercise is this: With quick step, firm hand, and limber finger, sprint to your telephone. Hoist up the receiver to your ear with a good grip. Insert your finger in the dial or dance over the buttons and call your doctor. You absolutely *must* make an appointment for a complete medical examination to do any of the exercises I do or any exercises that you might find anywhere.

You are not to read beyond this paragraph until you do this important exercise. If you do read beyond this point before you call your doctor, you will automatically gain four pounds.

Please do discuss these exercises and everything else in this book with your dear and glorious physician before you do anything more strenuous than lifting the phone.

BASICALLY LAZY

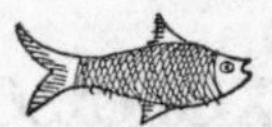

Fats Goldberg Sweats Or How A Kid Who Weighed 105 Pounds In The Third Grade, 240 Pounds In The Eighth Grade, And 265 Pounds In High School, Learned How To Throw A Baseball

Basically, I'm a lazy person. To me, sitting is the most underestimated pleasure of life. Give me a good seat at Yankee Stadium, or an aluminum-tubed plastic-webbed chair on a great beach, or a solid seat at a screaming horror movie, or a soft recliner in front of a TV set with a book, or a hard rocker with two close friends, and you'll find a happy man.

I like lying down but I go right to sleep when I lie down; there are only two things for me to do in bed. One of them is sleeping. Still, lying down beats standing. I'm not a big stander. I'm more of a leaner. If I stand in one place for over three minutes, I become a leaner. I can spot a comfortable automobile fender two blocks away.

EXERCISING REASON: HUFFIN', PUFFIN' TILL YOU'RE DOWN TO NOTHIN'!

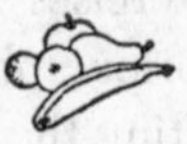

There are four reasons why I get my seat off the seat and exercise as much as I do.

1. Flat out, working out makes me feel terrific. Every tiny part of my body gets all tingly and juiced up. My energy level has shot up so much that if I sit too long in one place my legs start jerking and talking to me:

"Goldberg, come on, quit watching 'The Rockford Files.' Let's get going. We're not two skinny trees planted in this spot. We're falling asleep."

2. Moving around, flapping your arms up and down, or any physical messing around helps get rid of those sneaky, fiendish calories.

I swear I can see them parachuting out of the tips of my fingers, my toes, and through the large vacant acres between the hairs on my head.

3. Pushing my body around does great wonders for my heart and circulation.

4. Working out works all the lint and fuzz out of the mind.

Exercise is the Comet Cleaner of the head. One long walk gets rid of the bathtub ring of crazy notions, depressing thoughts, lost loves, and anything else that is clogging your brain.

School Days, School Days

Waddling out the back door of my house at the age of six or seven, I struggled over to the gym at Blessed Sacrament Catholic Church and School.

Those 100 short yards were some of the most important steps of my fat young life. The Catholic school system started their kids in organized sports at an age when I was still trying to get enough coordination to tie my shoes.

Growing up (and sideways) in a predominantly Catholic neighborhood, my pals were the McGlynns, Rogerses, Kellys, Saladinos, Lopezes, Andersons, and Rineharts.

All of them were hot jocks at the age of ten. For me to hang around with them, I had to rouse myself and get out there and play, too. What I really wanted to do was sit on the curb and eat Fudgsicles—but they wouldn't let me.

We played football, baseball, and basketball every free minute for years.

When I first started, I wasn't coordinated enough or strong enough to shoot the basketball and even hit the hoop. Plus when we chose up teams, I was always picked next to last. The only reason why I wasn't picked last was because of Patty McGlynn, a girl who was two years younger and sixty pounds lighter. Now that I think about it, she *was* picked ahead of me quite a few times.

Finally, after several months, I was actually running and playing for hours. But I didn't lose any weight. No sir. When it got dark and we had to go home for dinner, I hopped into Goldberg's Market like a famished, crazed kangaroo.

We played regardless of snow, rain, or heat straight through grade school, high school, and halfway through college.

Thanks to the other guys, the gym, and the tiny baseball field between the church and school, I developed coordination and strength. Without them, I probably couldn't even walk down the street without tripping.

Goldberg's Market

What also helped my coordination and strength was delivering groceries for Goldberg's Market, "Fancy Groceries and Meats, Free Delivery." (I was the free delivery.)

Sara and Art Goldberg had me on one of those Schwinn Cycle Trucks. You know, the bicycle with the big basket and small wheel on the front. I was hauling "Fancy Groceries and Meats" all over the hilly place. But I didn't lose weight riding that bike, either. Every time I came panting back from a delivery, it was a Mason's Root Beer and a Dolly Madison Banana Turnover.

Boy Scouts and Swimming

All right, so I'm not an Eagle Scout. But I am a Life Scout. I didn't get my Eagle Scout Badge because I was afraid of deep water and couldn't get Swimming and Life Saving merit badges.

Given the large surface area of my spongy body, though, I was a world champion floater.

But I sure do love the water and am a great shallow-water swimmer. I knew all the Life Saving strokes and carries. Still if I couldn't put my foot down and touch bottom, sheer panic would overcome my quivering form.

I'm forty-seven years old and still get teased about not being an Eagle Scout. I even called the Boy Scouts of America a couple of months ago to see if I could get my Eagle. They said I was a little too old: The maximum age is eighteen.

Golf and Caddying

Golf is one of my all-time favorite sports. I know people call it "barnyard pool" or "a pleasant little walk in the country." Still, there is something about hitting a good shot, and schlepping around a beautiful golf course is a tremendous experience.

I caddied for three years as a kid at Mission Hills Country Club in Kansas City. Used to make good bucks, too. I carried mostly "doubles"; one bag on each shoulder plus one pint of ice cream in each hand. With my weight, plus the weight of the golf bags, I developed muscles in my legs like a draft horse.

Tennis

Tennis always reminds me of standing on top of a huge Ping-Pong table. Who wants to do that?

Weight Lifting

Every guy I know lifted weights at one time or another. I used to lift weights every morning . . . raising 325 pounds out of my bed.

Gymnasiums and Health Spas

Too much hassle for me. I cannot get myself to go somewhere, rent a locker, unpack my plastic bag, put on my jock strap, $1.99 Woolworth shorts, T-shirt with a clever saying, 100 percent orlon tube socks, and holey sneakers and begin exercising with 150 other bodies.

All the exercising I do has to be worked into my normal life-style. I'd rather wear my regular clothes, in the privacy of my own home, and see the hysterical reaction of my own mirror. Why should total strangers have all the fun?

As for outdoor exercise, I'm a great believer in walking and running (more about these soon). And nobody laughs at runners and joggers anymore.

Stationary Bicycling

My doctor is a cardiologist, internist, and sausage-mushroom-onion pizza eater who prescribed stationary bicycling as one of the best exercises for fitness. Here was his prescription for me:

Take a fistful of bucks and buy a stationary bicycle with a

speedometer and a dial that allows for increase tension on the wheel. A timer is optional. You can always use your egg-splattered kitchen timer.

Eventually, after a preliminary program, I had to work up to the following level:

1. I must exercise every day. That's seven days a week.

2. I must exercise fifteen minutes every day.

3. I must pedal at a constant eighteen to twenty miles an hour. No faster.

4. I must get my pulse rate up to 120 beats per minute.

CAUTION WARNING CAUTION WARNING
CAUTION WARNING

This is what MY doctor told ME to do. You are an entirely different fitness person. If you want to start working out on a stationary bike, I must insist YOU GO TO YOUR DOCTOR and have him make out an exercise program and plan especially for you.

As I'm writing this on a Saturday morning, I just got off my bike, drank two glasses of water, and swallowed three tablespoons of raw bran.

The mileage on the speedometer reads 4,272 miles. I hadn't looked at it for a long time. Man, that's a long way. I think I'll go and lie down for a while.

THE NAKED KITCHEN

I planted my one-wheeled baby in the kitchen because it's the one room in my two and a half rooms that has the least action. I do my fifteen-minute ritual in the nude. My whole body breathes and it's more fun. If you get a stationary bicycle and want to pedal in the buff, I suggest you get a bike with a well-upholstered seat.

THE GOOD NEWS

When you exercise on a bike that goes nowhere, you can exercise any time you feel the twitch or sluggish, you can talk on the phone, you can move the bike out and start exercising in the backyard, terrace, or in the dining room while you're entertaining.

You can forget about thunderstorms, blizzards, cold, heat, dogs who attach themselves to your ankles, falling meteors, foot and knee problems, sunburn, and muggers.

THE BAD NEWS

Stationary bicycling is BORING, BORING, and BORING. I'm convinced boredom was invented on the stationary bicycle. It's about as exciting as runny vanilla ice milk.

Dr. Goldberg will now give you some personal remedies:

1. *Watching Television:* I climb on my bike between nine and ten in the morning. At nine, the Donahue Show comes on. Thank goodness for him. He's rescued me from boredom many mornings.

In New York now, we also can get "A.M. New York" or other talk shows in case Donahue has a lady sword swallower discussing her salt-free diet. Saturday mornings, I get to watch my favorite Bugs Bunny and Road Runner cartoons. Sunday morning means "Sunday Morning" with Charles Kuralt. One of the best programs anytime.

2. *Reading: People* magazine is perfect for two important events in my life.

The first is on a Cheating Day when I want a pepperoni-and-sausage pizza. I go in, make the pizza and throw it in the oven. By the time it bakes, I've eaten every strand of cheese and swigged two Cokes, I've read *People* and learned the latest gossip.

The second is that *People* is my pal on the bike. It has just the right reading consistency to make the time flow. I also get some screamingly funny quotes from Erik Estrada.

I even bought a reading stand for magazines and books that attaches to the handlebars.

3. *Daydreaming:* When nothing else works and those 900 seconds seem like eternity, I go into my Stationary Daydream Trance.

If that happens, there are no Super Bowls where I haven't caught the winning pass in the last five seconds; no unfriendly countries where I haven't been a dashing spy in my Burberry raincoat; no movie leading ladies I haven't romanced as I won my Oscar; no Broadway musical where I haven't stopped the show with my specialty number.

MORE GOOD NEWS

Hearing the bell go off, signaling the end of the fifteen minutes, I know I have the rest of the day made. My body is charged up, every cell is tingly, I feel terrific, and my heart is off to a good, pounding start.

TAKE A WALK

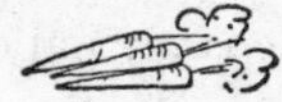

A Love Letter

My dearest darling Walking:

We first met in Chicago in 1959 where I was a dieting fat guy who thought a long walk was from my beige plastic chair to the refrigerator.

Then you tenderly took my hand and showed me Michigan Avenue, the Loop, Rush Street, Old Town, and, in the summer, the Oak Street Beach with the sand rushing between my toes and me staring at rows of beautiful women in bikinis. What an exciting world you opened to me.

In 1965, inflamed with love, you and I ran away to New York. Little did I know at the time, my sweet, that New York is one of the world's greatest Walking experiences.

How can I forget, even after all these lovely, blissful sixteen years with you, that there is a new street spectacular every ten feet; that walking boredom is unknown; that those concrete corridors beg to be trod by our cute Nike-shod feet; that our four- or five-mile daily schlep has kept me lean; that, without you, my love, my pants would still have a 48-inch waist.

What I admire about you is that you, Walking, are natural, no additives. Yes, humans were built to walk because we stand erect. Baby, we walk all the time.

You probably don't realize this about yourself, Silly, but walking is the best all-around exercise there is.

You love everyone; with no age barriers, old, young, and in-between can walk. And we can walk with you all our romantic lives. You even welcome folks with some disabilities who can benefit from your love.

Precious Walking, most anyone can do it. You demand no special training, clothes, or equipment, only comfortable walking shoes. I wear running shoes to move more quickly beside you. The weather doesn't stop us either. What you are is a cheap passionate date, every man's dream.

But our most fun date is when we meet friendly women, neighbors, nice dogs, planning our Controlled Cheating Day, learning about our neighborhood, and making new pals and lovers everywhere.

You're so adaptable and giving, Sweetheart. We can work you into any of our strange life-styles. We can walk to work, walk to lunch, walk after dinner, walk to the store. Walk, walk, walk, you darling little fool.

Ha, Angel, you do have your little regulations, don't you? We must walk briskly at the rate of three miles an hour for thirty minutes a day. And we should walk with a steady rhythm, breathing deeply and swinging our arms. You always remind us that when we get tired we should sit down and rest before going on.

Plus, Light of My Life, we must be consistent and walk every day, maybe taking the whole family along or walking with a friend or friends.

Walking, you're so good for us physically and mentally. We sleep better and walking improves circulation, blood to the heart, and helps reduce blood pressure. You also help us build muscle strength. Nervous? Tense? Troubled? Take a walk and clear the brain.

Sweet Patootie, you're so wonderful for folks who are flabby, out of shape, or non-athletic. You won't hurt us like other exercises that are so strenuous.

My favorite times with you, Devoted One, is when we eat and walk at the same time. Funny me. I know it burns up calories.

After eating is also one of my favorite times with you. Time for using up more of those ugly little calories.

Buttercup, you probably don't know this about yourself, but if a 150-pound person walks for an hour, four days a week, at three miles an hour, they will lose about twelve pounds a year, if they eat the same amount of food as they did before walking. If they eat less then they'll lose even more weight.

Honey Bunch, Snookums, I must tear myself away from you now.

We shall meet again in about thirty minutes when you and I will walk to the Gaiety Delicatessen for brunch.

I miss you already, Heart of Hearts.

You will always be my Perfect "10" in the exercise department.

XOXOXOXOXOXOXOXOXOXOX
Fats

YOGA

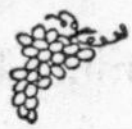

Every morning for the last twenty years, I have hauled an old yellow hunk of foam rubber out of the closet and done three yoga "postures." I yoga before I climb on the stationary bicycle.

The Shoulder Stand

I started this five-minute daily ritual because in one of the 4,283,912 diet and exercise books I've read it said that we all should have one "inversion" a day. This means that we should get our feet higher than our head, which lets the blood nourish the brain. The poor old brain sits up there all the time and it needs an extra shot of the plasma.

Besides, I also read that a daily inversion is good for the hair department. The same blood that helps out the brain can also nourish the hair follicles. I think it works.

1. Lie flat on your back, arms at your sides. Your hands are next to your thighs, palms down.

2. Palms gripping the floor, tense the abdomen and legs as you slowly allow your legs to rise to a ninety-degree angle (or as close as you can get to it).

3. Use your hands to prop your hips up in the air as your legs swing back toward your head.

4. Straighten your legs and back so that they are at a ninety-degree angle to your head. The head and shoulders take all the weight. Keep your chin pressed to your chest to relieve any strain on your neck. Be controlled, relaxed but not rigid.

5. Try to hold the position for three minutes. When you are ready to come down, do so slowly and carefully, always in controlled movements, never sudden or jerky. Relax the legs, bending the knees toward the forehead, and lower carefully. Use the hands, palms down for support. When the legs touch the floor, turn palms upward and relax.

The Alternate Leg Pull

This is a wonderful stretching exercise for the legs, back, and stomach.

1. Sit on the floor, both legs straight out in front of you.

2. Take hold of the right foot with both hands, bend the right knee, and draw the foot up until the sole is resting against the inside of the left thigh.

3. Reach the arms toward the ceiling and lean backward slightly, inhaling deeply.

4. Exhale, using the breath to help bring your body forward, and grasp your left leg at the furthest point you can without strain.

If you can't reach your ankle, try for the calf or the knee. Keep the knee as close to the floor as you can. Do not bend the leg to reach further—that defeats the point of the stretch. It's okay to bend the elbows though. That helps lower the torso. The stretch should be held for thirty seconds.

5. Sit up, releasing your grasp, switch the left foot to the right thigh, and repeat as above. Do each leg two times.

The longer you practice the leg pulls, the more flexible you'll become. You'll be able to reach further down the leg. Eventually you'll be able to clasp your foot. This is the advanced position. When you can grab your foot—or even extend your hands past your soles—add the following for a really terrific leg, back, and torso stretch:

a. After repeating steps 1–3 above, as you reach forward grasp the foot in your hands.

b. Relax your neck, send the elbows outward, and aim your forehead toward your knee. Stay there for thirty seconds.

c. Release the foot and come up slowly to the original sitting position. Repeat with the other leg.

The Cobra

No, I do not keep a pet snake around to exercise with. The Cobra is a very powerful yoga posture that's very beneficial for the back.

1. Lie flat on your tummy, forehead touching the floor, arms at your sides, palms up. Relax into the floor.

2. Very sloooowly inhale and raise the forehead, the nose, and the chin. This tilts the head back. Continue arching the neck, the shoulders, and the back.

3. Place the hands palm down on the floor directly below the shoulders and lean on them to help raise the body even higher, continually arching back until only the hands, abdomen, and legs touch the floor. Straighten the arms as you raise more of the body up. With practice, you'll be able to raise the entire torso. Hold for a count of ten.

4. Exhale, bringing the body back down slowly, bending the elbows to help lower first the abdomen, the shoulders, the chin, nose, and the forehead last. Place the arms at your sides and relax. Do three times.

Running Up and Down the Stairs

Climbing up and down stairs for the last ten years has been a rough, tough physical conditioner that is a great exerciser for the legs and heart. I started walking very slowly for only three flights. That's when I lived on the fifth floor. After a few months, I was hustling all the way up and down five.

Eight years ago I moved to the seventh floor and cautiously worked on going up to six flights and then finally to seven.

Now I quickly walk up and down those ninety-eight steps, even if I do pant at the top. I do those seven fun-filled flights five or six times a day.

Gang, I don't like those stairs at all, but like it or not, I set my firm jaw, grit my teeth, and start marching.

I rarely take the elevator unless I'm carrying my laundry bag or a big watermelon.

Sometimes when the elevator door is open, I longingly stick my big toe in, but I quickly jerk it out again. Not only because the elevator door is making an accordion of my leg, but I feel I owe it to my body to climb.

Mount Everest must be easier than this.

Jogging

What can I say about an exercise where millions of folks slip on flimsy underwear, use $60 shoes that weigh two ounces, are outside in monsoons and volcanic eruptions, work their hearts out, and have twenty different magazines to explain what they're doing?

What do I say? I say jogging is terrific. I don't do a whole lot of jogging. In fact, I only jog in the dead of winter when it's cold enough to make my down jacket quack. I run to keep me warm as I travel. I wear cheap running shoes and various-colored Levi's all the time anyway. So I leap out on the sidewalk that's the temperature of an iceberg and start moving. With all the strange and wonderful walkers on the streets of New York, sometimes my jogging is more like a walk on the wild side.

The Pittsburgh Steelers could use me as a swivel-hipped half-back, dodging gaunt fashion models carrying gaunt briefcases, white-faced mimes who are trying to be the next Mork, shopping bag ladies, those steaming hot dog and pretzel carts (sauerkraut, onions, *and* mustard, please), and twitching advertising salesmen who just dropped $165 for lunch at the Four Seasons.

A half mile or ten blocks of running is about all I can manage at one time. I'm telling you, by the time the first city-hardened robin nests on my dirty old air conditioner, I'm in great shape and feel sensational.

Walking will always be number one with me. But I'd also like to become sort of a regular jogger. About fifteen or twenty minutes a day would do it. Nothing too strenuous; only enough to get my corns to stand at attention.

Putting on special funny clothes, going to a special funny

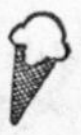

Vacation Cheating and Non-Cheating

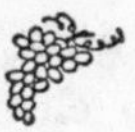

C.H.E.A.T. The Congress of Healthy Eating All the Time New Union Contract Concerning Vacations, Cheating, Non-Cheating, and Having Seven Full Days Off Twice a Year. The Union Meeting to be held on The Good Ship Lollipop.

"Attention. May I have your attention, please. Will the members tear themselves away from the salad bar and please find seats. There are plenty of good seats in the front. I won't bite you, unless I get really hungry.

"First, the membership would like to welcome the new members, The Goal Weighters, who have served their diet apprenticeship and are now entitled to all benefits and privileges accorded the beloved membership of the C.H.E.A.T. Union.

"As your President, Cuisine Art, I must tell you that we have had some problems in the bread Board Room during the negotiations with the Executive Board and certain Shop Stewards.

"I hate to report to the membership that Sara Lee punched

out the Pillsbury Dough Boy. Chef Boyardee resigned as vice president in charge of ravioli. Arthur Treacher proposed marriage to Ann Page, who promptly hit him in the face with one of her pumpkin pies. Ronald McDonald and Burger King are still not speaking, due to both being in love with Wendy's Hot and Juicy Hamburgers. Colonel Sanders stormed out in a huff, when we ordered in fried chicken from Brown's Chicken. Other than these insignificant problems, everything went as smooth as Dannon Lemon Yogurt.

"There is one sad announcement. Irving Shakey of Shakey's Pizza is retiring from active membership. He and the missus will be retiring to Hershey, Pennsylvania, where they will try to invent a chocolate anchovy. Irving wanted me to tell all of you he'd sure be pleased if you'd stop by and see them in Hershey. The missus said they'd always have a bed for you in an abandoned pizza oven. Irving, as one of our Charter Members, we're going to miss you.

"On to the terms of the Vacation Contract with Fats Goldberg and his Controlled Cheating Corporation. We have done some hard, heavy bargaining that went non-stop for six and a half months. The Executive Committee, the Shop Stewards (when they weren't fighting), and I have come up with what we think is a fair proposal from Fats Goldberg concerning our rights to eat on vacations.

"Will the Sergeant of Arms, Dairy Queen, please pass out copies of the new Vacation Contract. There is one negative note. Due to inflation there will be a Tastee Freez on wages."

VACATIONS: THE C.H.E.A.T. UNION CONTRACT

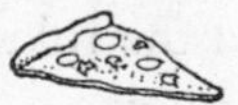

(To be posted at all water fountains, soda and candy machines, or anywhere that calories are dispensed.)

Article One:

You May Control Cheat Seven Consecutive Days Twice A Year.

Rejoice and celebrate. Applaud yourself. Your new contract says you now can have seven uninterrupted Controlled Cheating days twice a year. VACATION!

Every morning, your happy eyes open like pistachio nuts and stare at the candy-striped pillow case. A big grin sweeps across your face getting a mouth full of candy-striped lint. You know you can eat that day and every day for the next seven triumphant days.

It makes no difference whether you're sleeping under the stars in your camper in West Texas, under silk sheets in The Carlyle Hotel in New York City, under a blinking no-vacancy sign at a Ramada Inn in Santa Barbara, California, or waking up under your own roof in Arlington Heights, Illinois; you, Controlled Cheater, are on vacation.

What a combination. A well-deserved rest from work and a well-served Cheating Eating Vacation. The best two weeks of your year!

This is some big eating deal for you. But like all good union contracts there are certain key provisions that *MUST* be followed to stay in compliance with Fats Goldberg and The Controlled Cheating Corporation.

You are a valued member of the organization and we would

be totally lost without you. Your diet productivity and personality are essential to the success of the Company. Besides, you bake dynamite walnut brownies. You are indispensable. We need you back so please read the rules and regulations carefully for your Cheating Eating Vacations.

Provision: Goal Weight

No Controlled Cheater may go on a Seven-Day Consecutive Cheating Vacation until they have been at Goal Weight for AT LEAST THREE MONTHS.

You know as well as I do why that rule is in the contract. I want you to be completely comfortable in your new Goal Weight life. So content and easy with Controlled Cheating that you'll be able to go back on your diet as easily as you would slip on your favorite maroon felt carpet slippers.

Seven hot days of good-time eating is one heck of a lot of goodies. You're a professional Controlled Cheater after all these months. Being the Boss Eater, I have confidence in your reliability. You will return to the Cheating Eating assembly line with renewed vigor and snapshots of the meals you ate.

Provision: You May *Not* Cheat Fourteen Days in a Row on Your Vacation

Let's go over that again. You may NOT, under any silly circumstances, reasons, excuses, or alibis whatever, cheat for two straight weeks. Talk about blowing your whole diet. This would be it. Taking a two-weeks-in-a-row eating vacation is as risky as going to dinner at a skinny couple's home where they serve Cheez Whiz on Ritz Crackers instead of the salad.

If I let you take fourteen days of cheating, you'd be down that fat road faster than Al Unser at the Indianapolis 500.

You've worked too hard to blow it all at once. I tried two straight weeks of eating about fifteen years ago. It took everything I had to get back to my Goal Weight. I'll talk about that later.

Once more, for the delayed broadcast to the West Coast: You may not take your two-week Cheating Eating Vacation in one huge gulp. One week at a time is it.

Provision: No Bozo Eating

Look, you know all there is to know about bozo or crazy eating. You've educated yourself from your Controlled Cheating Days. We'll go over nutsy eating just once more because it's vitally important in your Seven-Straight-Day Eating Vacation: *Only eat when you're hungry and only eat foods you truly crave.*

Planning is as important for these seven days as the cone is to ice cream. You're looking at seven straight days of big time, high-level dining. That's 168 hours of fun twice a year.

Make sure you eat a whole variety of good foods. Go to places you didn't have time for on your regular Controlled Cheating Days. Nosh your way around town, like I do in New York. Or have a barbecue at home. Do anything and everything you want in the eating department. But use your imagination: Don't fool around with no-fun, no-flavor washouts like white bread, American cheese, and miniature marshmallows.

Provision: How to Cheat and Diet When You Are Gone for Two Weeks or Longer on Vacation

1. You must stick to your normal cheating every third day the First Week and Cheat the Second Week, Not the Other Way around. If you cheat the first week of your vacation and try to diet the second, the Las Vegas odds on you are 1,000 to 1 that you won't stop cheating the second week.

It's going to be tougher than nickel steak for you not to cheat the first week of your vacation, even if you planned to diet that first week. But you must stick to it!

But if you actually plan to cheat the first week of your vacation and diet the second, I'm standing here eyeball to eyeball telling you that you're going to cheat for fourteen straight days. This will be a *disaster* and jeopardize your whole Controlled Cheating Program.

Unless you always dreamed of being a kamikaze pilot in World War II, DO NOT DO IT!

2. *How to Diet on Vacations* Dieting while you're running around the U.S. or the world is exactly the same as when you're at home except you have to be even more careful for many reasons.

First, the pizza and popsicles you eat in Hollywood, California, have the same amount of corrupting calories as the pizza and popsicles in Hollywood, Florida.

Second, you're eating in a different hot spot for almost every meal. This is difficult because you don't know how each fixes their Blue Plate Specials. Make sure everything is baked, broiled, or boiled. No fried foods. Remember that fried foods have twice as many calories as the same foods baked, broiled, or boiled.

Many places offer a low-calorie or diet plate, too. Don't eat the crackers or little cellophane packages of wafers they always stick on the side of the plate. That's pure bozo!

I always try to order "natural" foods. When I say natural, I'm not talking about foods from one of those quaint health food stores with the fake Tiffany lamps, high prices, and a salesman who looks like he just got out of solitary confinement in a Turkish prison. Natural, to me, means foods the guy behind the counter with the greasy apron and toothpick hanging out of his mouth is not likely to mess around with (for instance, fresh fruits like cantaloupe, grapefruit, apples, and bananas). Also, individual cans of water-packed tuna fish instead of tuna salad where they might add a quart of mayo. I want to cut out "hidden" calories that are added to the point where you might as well go and have a Big Mac.

When I go into an unfamiliar café, I study the menu like I'm looking for a secret message from the C.I.A. that will solve the Mid-East Crisis.

If the menu looks like I'm in serious trouble, I'll order a dry salad with a wedge of fresh lemon for the dressing, being careful not to swallow the seeds, and a baked potato with no butter or sour cream. The baked potato has only about ninety calories without all the extra stuff and it's very filling.

When you do order something like chicken, shrimp, or tuna salad sandwich, ask for it "off" the bread. Then you'll get the salad squatting on the plate all by itself with maybe a little lettuce and tomato.

Third, do your best to stay away from fast-food restaurants. If your family or friends insist, stamp your feet, pout, laugh and cry at the same time, and hysterically roll your eyes round and round. Okay, this doesn't work. Go in and order a sandwich, take off the bread (it's usually tasteless and gummy anyway), order a diet soda, and afterward don't say a word for thirteen straight hours or until they buy you a juicy Red Delicious apple.

Fourth, psychologically you must be stronger. You're out of your home turf. At home you know exactly what you are doing and what you're going to eat. Plus you can leap at the refrigerator to get a fresh peach when the dieting gets tough.

What else can I tell you, Controlled Cheater? Use your good diet sense and the experience you've had these many months and above all have a good vacation and don't worry, I'll be here when you get back.

Provision: Eating on the Run, or Controlled Cheat Dining in Public Transportation and Your Own Car

AIRPLANE EATING

Everyone laughs and makes fun of the food served on airplanes. It's always good for a few snickers from your bored friends who have a few hilarious airline food stories of their own. We've all had the beige Salisbury steaks, pink cake, and pitted peas on Flight 99 nonstop from Lima to Columbus, Ohio.

The good news is that most airlines offer us serious Controlled Cheaters a big selection of low-calorie and special meals along with their astronomical fare prices.

Here are just a few of the dietetic and special meals you can order. You must ask for a special meal at least twenty-four hours in advance or preferably when you make your reservation.

1. Low-calorie or Dietetic
2. Cold Seafood Platter (only certain airlines have this one)
3. Vegetarian
4. Low-sodium or Salt-free.

SHIPS, TRAINS, AND BUSES

Ships: The only large object that I've been to sea with that floats was my old 325-pound body. The only big boat I've ever been on was the Circle Line Cruise boat around the island of Manhattan where they serve terrible hot dogs and great frozen custard.

What I hear from folks who go on grown-up cruises for their vacations is that a ship is a dieter's nightmare. It's nonstop feeding from early morning until late at night with snacks in between.

Sorry, you're going to have to tooth-check ships yourself. Be very, very careful.

Trains and Buses: Bring a Sears shopping bag with your own goodies.

CAR CUISINE

The automobile and I have had an eating love affair for all my born days. There have been seven beautiful cars in my past. The first was sold to me by two of my uncles, Jimmy and Harry, who owned A-to-Z Auto Wrecking. They pulled a 1937 Oldsmobile from the pile and gave it to me for $30. It was love at first sight. But my baby had a problem. Every time I stopped, all the oil in the motor leaked out on the ground. No one would let me park in their driveways. All my money went for food and oil.

Twice a week I had to sweep out the floors of the front and back because of the build-up of watermelon seeds, Dolly Madison cake wrappers, carmel corn, and crumbs from cheeseburgers.

The last car I bought was a 1960 Volkswagen that I sold in 1965 when I moved from Chicago to New York. That baby was an insurance policy for me when I went from 325 pounds to 190 in 1959. The sun roof car cost $1,812 with push-button radio and white walls and was a great incentive to stay skinny. If I put on two pounds, I'd never be able to fit in the front seat again.

My eyes glaze over with tears of eating happiness when I think about all the delicious groceries I've devoured in the seats and on the running boards of those seven three-ton rolling lunch boxes.

Give me a car and a highway and I start daydreaming of roadside burger joints, soft ice cream, and the one and only, best eating of them all, gas stations. Yeah, gas stations. They have a limited menu, the service is fast, and the food is cheap.

My love affair with dining in gas stations started when I was growing up on Thirty-ninth and Agnes in Kansas City. There were two gas stations across the street.

One was a Texaco station owned by the Meyers Brothers. The candy machine had only a fair selection. It was heavy on packages of peanut butter spread on orange-colored crackers. The Coke machine was a treat and had not only Coke but Mission Orange and Mason's Root Beer.

The other station was a Phillips 66 owned by my cousin, Dave. The Coke machine was so-so with only Coke, 7-Up, and Grapette. The candy machine was okay. What they did have was a one-cent peanut machine that gave you a handful of the saltiest, greasiest peanuts in the world.

I'm going to give you one of the only two recipes I know in the whole world. The first is for all kinds of pizzas.

This is the other one:

1. Take one ice-cold bottle of Coca-Cola, a bottle, not a can.

2. Gulp down two large swigs.

3. Get the greasiest, saltiest peanuts you can buy, preferably with the red skins still on.

4. Take a medium handful of peanuts and pour them in the Coke bottle. You can lick the palm of your hand for the extra salt.

Take a gurgle of Coke and peanuts and start chewing that heavenly mixture of Coke, peanuts, salt, and grease. You might never come back to earth.

I can't take any more of this excitement. I'm going to take a cold shower.

Dieting in cars, campers, trailers, or anything else that rolls on highways or dirt roads is easy on vacations. You and the Dalton Gang in the back seat are a self-contained unit. No goodies can come in except those that you buy and put on the seat.

All those roadside eateries do reach out their yummy paws

and want to drag you in. But you have the flexibility to roar on down that road.

When I used to have a car and drive and diet, I'd always have a big bag of fruit in the front seat next to me. I could reach in and whip out a peach, apple, plum, or anything else. My sticky steering wheel smelled like a fruit cocktail.

There are also advantages in diet highway eating. You can stop at roadside farm stands and buy fresh-picked vegetables direct from the field that's twelve feet away. There's absolutely nothing better than a fresh-picked home-grown tomato that you eat like an apple.

When you stop for gas, stay in the car. Don't mosey around the station looking in the goody machines unless it's a Controlled Cheating Day.

Another advantage of dieting in an automobile is that gas is so high you won't have any extra money to eat anyway.

Provision: You Must Leave Your Scale at Home

Leave that baby on the bathroom floor. When I say vacation, I mean vacation from everything, including the tyranny and twitchiness of hopping on the scale every morning.

There are times I wanted to take my scale with me on vacations. I thought I'd buy a velvet-lined scale satchel from Samsonite for easy carrying. They haven't invented one yet. But I stifled the urge, kissed my Health-O-Meter good-bye, locked the door, and happily danced down the stairs, free at last.

Provision: You Must Go Back on Your Diet After Vacation

You are going to panic. I know because I've panicked every six months for the last twenty-two years. The panic attacks you the moment you open your eyes the morning after the Seven Days of Controlled Cheating.

Panic Button #1: This button pushes that part of your mind that says, "How in the world can I go back on that awful low-calorie balanced diet after I've had seven fun-filled days of uninterrupted eating? I'm going to stay under these covers the rest of my life."

Off Button #1: You can turn Panic Button #1 off because you only have six short days of dieting before you can cheat again. That's SIX DAYS of low-calorie balanced dieting. After those six days, you have your regular Cheating Eating Day. Then it's back to your Every Third Day Program. Once more, that is SIX DAYS OF DIETING before you can cheat again. Dream back over your Eating Vacation and relive those Magic Masticating Moments.

All right chorus, let's hear your old favorite hymn. First the sopranos, then the altos and basses, you come right in. Ready?

"I Must Go Back on My Diet." Sing that song again.

"I MUST GO BACK ON MY DIET." Solid!

Panic Button #2: After you crawl out of bed and after you turn off Panic Button #1, you must weigh yourself.

Yes, you must stand up straight, look dead ahead, and resolutely walk to where your scale is hiding. Without any fuss, climb up on your scale and look directly down at the dial. No hesitating.

Off Button #2: Before you step up on the scale, turn on the shower, radio, or television full force. This will drown out your whimpers, cries, or screams without bothering the rest of the family.

After you've gotten that out of your system, you'll be fine. Who cares what that dumb dial says? You had a great seven days. You planned it all out, so there is no guilt or depression. You knew exactly what you were doing every step of the way. AND, there are only six small days until you can Control Cheat again.

Don't expect the scale dial to go right back to your Goal Weight (the weight you were before you went on vacation) in six days. That is going to take time. But over a period of weeks your weight will gradually return to your Goal Weight. Above all, don't skip any Cheating Days. You still need them.

You'll probably even be glad to get back on your diet, because you feel so much better when you're lighter.

I sure wish there was some other way to do this but . . . after you get back from Seven Straight Days of Controlled Cheating,

YOU MUST GO BACK ON YOUR DIET!
YOU MUST GO BACK ON YOUR DIET FOR SIX STRAIGHT DAYS! THEN YOU MAY HAVE A CHEATING EATING DAY. AFTER THAT IT IS BACK TO YOUR EVERY THIRD DAY EATING PROGRAM!

"I think we have a terrific contract here. Let's vote. Everybody in favor, yell CHOCOLATE. Everybody opposed, yell CELERY.

"Since no one yelled celery and the scream for chocolate was shattering, the new contract passes unanimously.

"Meeting adjourned."

Eats Side
Wets Side
All Around the Town

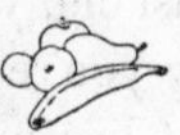

You've come a long way, baby, with your regular routine of Controlled Cheating and dieting. Hold on. I want to be especially careful that no Big Event or Swank Soiree comes along that will throw you over the side of your Good Ship Lollipop to the always lurking hungry UNcontrolled Cheating sharks.

Many folks, like you, feel hunger-crazed butterflies soaring in the region of your body you know best—just behind your darling belly button. This tummy twitching comes from Big Deal Dining Out.

Your friendly neighborhood Goldcheater is here to put cool compresses against your fevered brow and say, never you fret. After waltzing through this whole program of Controlled Cheating so smoothly, you're not about to succumb to nervousness.

Heck, you've already proven to yourself day after day that you've been able to take control over a mighty important part of your life—eating. What you can do around your own pink Formica kitchen table, you can do in front of new folks, large luminaries, and romantic encounters.

DINING OUT ON A CHEATING DAY

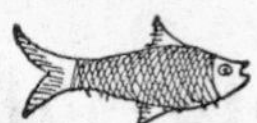

Try to be the one to make the arrangements when you must eat out. Then you can make the date on one of your Cheating Days. There's no sense in spending a lot or even a little money on a Diet Day. You'll have more laughs when you can cheat legitimately and enjoy the goodies. When the other folks are doing the asking, you have to go along with them. Soon enough they'll know you're a Controlled Cheater and will ask you out on your next Cheating Day.

That is very kind of them and shows they care. Why don't you introduce me?

Boredom

Boredom in any eatery is dangerous for us. You can't run away; you can't start reading *Mad* magazine; you have to sit there where your idle little hands can pick up little French fries from someone else's plate and slide them into your rosebud mouth, which then won't be idle.

My favorite cure for boredom, when you're not having a good time, is to take a peaceful cruise into your imagination. Think about a specific problem you want to solve: like her fake fingernail fell off and is sitting on top of her coconut sherbet. Or you can dream about you and Barbra Streisand starring in *The Weight We Were*. Or better yet, daydream what you're going to eat on your next Controlled Cheating Day.

BIG BIZ, SOCIAL, AND DATING EATS

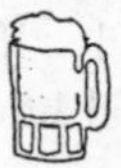

Big Biz, social, and dating eats I've stuck together because we all have to go out and meet new people, and eat in restaurants and houses where there are mounds of goodies just waiting for us to run through barefoot. What I'm trying to tell you is that I also get nervous in these situations.

I know that I must double my mighty resolve to keep my little link sausage fingers from dancing across the table to spear a handful of pasta.

Low-calorie balanced eating at a business lunch or dinner is easier than parties-and-dating eating. You're on business to talk over the sale of your newest product, Acme Inflatable Two-Strap T-shirts. You're too busy talking and threatening. If you're not talking, you can always make pictures in the tablecloth with your fork or hide behind your Diet Pepsi can.

Dating Eats

Lunch dates are a terrific way to get to know a new sweetie pie. Your time is limited. The lunch menu is usually cheaper than the dinner menu. And if either one of you suddenly discover that you'd rather be sitting in a dentist's chair than being there, you can always say, "I have to run back to work." Beware, eating hysterics are still possible regardless of how short the lunch.

Dinner dates are open ended, meaning hours of being charming, witty, on your best behavior, and worst of all, dressed up. I'm always afraid my tie will hang in the chocolate mousse.

Never tell your friend you're on a diet. That will make them twitchy. Remember, don't be a Diet Bore. You can show off to yourself and prove how good a Controlled Cheater you are.

On dates, eat verrrry slooowly. If you don't, the meal will be over in eight minutes and you'll have to go somewhere else and spend more money. Forget what your mother said about not playing with your food. Messing around with your plate will make you slow down to a crawl. This will also give the other person the impression that you're so absorbed and entranced with them that you can barely eat.

Neil Simon couldn't have produced a better setting for sticking your buttered thumb in a soft pumpernickel and raisin roll and licking it like a Fudgsicle. Especially if the conversation is running down to the point where you've asked her where she went to school for the third time in six minutes. The important thing is to relax. You've proven to yourself that you're a dynamite Controlled Cheater and that nothing can make you cheat. Have a good time.

Who Picks? Who Pays?

Business eating is expense account stuff, so go to town, dietwise. "Damn the expense, full low calories ahead," unless there is a maximum that your boss gives you to spend, and you want to hold on to your job past four-thirty on the afternoon when he's checking expense accounts.

Social and dating is another can of home-baked pork and beans. I like the very moderate café that could even be called cheap. Unless, of course, my gorgeous date is paying her fair share. Then we can go anywhere.

Women's Lib is here to stay. Any guy in his right mind has to go for it all . . . including the liberated woman who forks over for her share of the eats.

My big problem is how to tell the lady I'm asking that I want her to pay for her end of the date. Shoot. The women I take out make as much or more than I do. It's only fair that they pay their own freight. Right? Darn right! No wonder I can't get a date.

ROUTE EATY-EAT

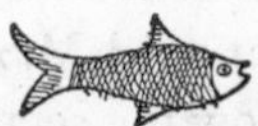

Route Eaty-Eat is the big white cottage cheese highway with the fresh pineapple median strip that takes you on a scenic dietetic schlep through the beautiful sky-high mountains of Expensive Beaneries, along breathtaking plains of middle of the roadhouses, and then plunges down and weaves through the deep dish valleys of Cheap Eateries.

Using your Controlled Cheating Reducing Roadmap, you can negotiate any dangerous curves and get a low-cal meal at any number of roadside diners and truck stops.

Expensive Beaneries

In my limited experience with Big Buck Beaneries, I've found it's easy to get a terrific low-calorie, balanced meal. There is plenty of fish, chicken, and lean meat on the menu. The fancily dressed chef will cook it any way you want and the portions are smaller.

Thinking about expensive restaurants, I don't remember seeing many heavy people dining. It must be when you're eating custom-cooked foods with the finest ingredients, you don't need as much to eat.

But when they roll that dessert cart over to the table you roll under the table with your Red Delicious apple.

Middle of the Roadhouses

Veer into any coffee shop, café, restaurant, or delicatessen. You can order turkey, tuna, chicken, roast beef, broiled fish, clear chicken consommé, mixed green salads, fresh fruit, plus many of these places offer special dietetic plates.

Chinese and Japanese truck stops are terrific for the slim traveler. Most everything is custom cooked. So you can tell them to cut out the butter, salt, sugar, and M.S.G. Also they're very big on chicken and fish. They know the secret of slimness.

Almost every eatery now has a salad bar. If you're not careful you can load up with enough calories so that you might just as well have ordered a triple cheeseburger, fries, chocolate shake, and a slice of apple pie a la mode.

You've got to stay away from the huge vats of salad dressings, bacon bits, cheese, and anything else that looks like it could make you and the dial quiver when you get on the scale the next morning.

Cheap Eateries

You know by now that the writer is one of the cheapest human beings who ever asked for a doggie bag for the boney end of a chicken wing.

I've made finding low-calorie restaurants a game. You can, too, regardless of where you live. There are many fine cheap cafés everywhere. Look for small Chinese and Japanese and other oriental places that are run by families: low overhead, low prices. In fact, look for small Mom-and-Pop operations of any description; they aim to please. Besides, looking for good cheap cafés that serve some low-cal dishes can be fun. You could even write a guide book.

You know you're going to end up at a lot of burger, chicken,

folds and ten belts (none of them fit because the givers, of course, underestimated the girth of a thirteen-year-old kid) and I saw a movie that changed my life. The movie was *The Lost Weekend* with Ray Milland and Jane Wyman. Ray got an Academy Award for his performance and Jane got Ronald Reagan. Billy Wilder directed and co-wrote.

Don't miss it when it comes on the Late Show. It's the story of an alcoholic writer and his plunge into the depths of sickness, poverty, and hallucinations. And that's only the happy parts.

When I walked out of that movie, I was in a daze. *The Lost Weekend* literally cured my drinking problem before I ever tasted hard liquor. I didn't realize it at the time, though.

The first time I ever drank hard whiskey was in September 1954 in the hot humid basement of the Zeta Beta Tau fraternity house at the University of Missouri. I got loaded. Boy, did I have a great time for about fifty-seven minutes. Then I stumbled upstairs and had my head in the wash basin for the next two days.

Getting roaring drunk was a Saturday night ritual for about two months. I'd start slow and end up swigging out of the bottle. Then I'd spend the rest of Saturday night and all day Sunday in the third stall of the toilet.

One of the reasons I drank was to give me enough courage to try and "make out" with a little A E Phi cutie I was laveliered to. You got it. This didn't work either. We'd walk back to her sorority house, go up the stairs to the door, and I'd get ready for action. She stopped. I made my move. Nothing. A little peck on my pouty lips and she'd bolt upstairs.

One Saturday night we were sitting there in the basement with the rest of the gang. Everything was as usual; one bottle of scotch and two dirty water glasses and my little sweetie.

I looked at that jug of whiskey and I said to myself, "This stuff tastes horrible. What am I doing? It tastes awful, I get sick as a dog, and I don't make out anyway." That's when I decided not to drink anymore. Sure, since 1954 I've been drunk a couple of more times. But it's been about fifteen years now since I've even had a taste of whiskey.

Liquor tasted to me like medicine. I was used to soda, ice cream malts, and sweet things. Drinking was stupid for me, for two reasons. I sure wasn't enjoying the taste. And I had terminal nausea and hangovers. Let me tell you when a 280-pounder has a hangover, that's a severe problem.

What other folks do is fine with me. I can sit in bars, go to parties or anywhere else where there's drinking and have tomato juice, diet soda, or plain water.

Getting down to the nitty-gritty, I have enough problems with food addiction without bringing in other stuff.

Goldberg's Saloon

Controlled Cheater, belly up to the bar, plant your tootsies on the brass rail, hunker down, put both elbows on the varnish, and I'll buy you a drink.

"THE EYEBALL SOUR"

A very tart drink. When you and your pals sit down, they order whiskey, wine, and beer and you order Tab with lemon. They start cajoling and teasing you about not drinking. What they're actually saying is they think you're making a moral judgment about them—which you are not. Tell your friends the truth. I say, "I don't like the taste." Your truth could be, "I don't want to blow the calories," or "I get too hungry when I drink," or "I only drink wine made from a very rare grape, The Angela Lans Berry." When you sip, beautiful singing fills your body.

"FROSTY ALTERNATIVE"

What DO you order if everyone else is sitting around the Dew Drop Inn? Here is a cocktail you can make any number of ways. Some of them are:

I stick to diet soda with lemon; regular soda "on the rocks"; plain tomato juice (also known as a "Virgin Mary"); plain orange juice (never heard a clever name for this one; maybe it should be called a "Virgin Driver"); plain club soda, "straight up"; or, of course, the elegant imported waters in funny-looking bottles. I personally refuse to pay a buck and a half for six ounces of plain water with fizz in it, regardless of what fancy foreign spring it shoots out of. Here's the Cheapo Goldberg Alternative, plain tap water. You can order it "on the rocks, straight up, or with a twist." And best of all it's free, with NO calories.

ALCOHOL "CALORIE COUNTER"

Alcohol actually gives you knowledge when you drink it. These highballs speak to you about how many calories they have. Put your ear to the rim of the glass and they'll tell you many secrets. Listen.

	CALORIES
Beer: One 12-ounce can or bottle (4.5 percent alcohol by volume)	151
Gin, Rum, Vodka, Whiskey	
80-proof: Jigger 1½ fluid ounces	97
86-proof: Jigger 1½ fluid ounces	105
90-proof: Jigger 1½ fluid ounces	110
94-proof: Jigger 1½ fluid ounces	116
100-proof: Jigger 1½ fluid ounces	124
Wines	
Dessert (18.8 percent alcohol by volume)	
Wine glass (serving portion 3½ fluid ounces)	141

	CALORIES
Table (12.2 percent alcohol by volume)	
Wine glass (serving portion 3½ fluid ounces)	87

These figures come from the U. S. Department of Agriculture Handbook No. 456, "Nutritive Value of American Foods."

THIS IS WAR!!!

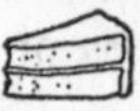

The Battlefield: Any holiday, party, outdoor barbecue, pal's dinner party, relatives' roundup, picnic, soiree, wedding, or any mob scene of more than two but less than 20,000 people where there is the ENEMY: the dreaded Army of Fattening Foods on a Non-Cheating Day.

The Soldier: You, Controlled Cheater. Women and men are both drafted in this person's army. Both have to be on the front lines ready to do battle with the ENEMY.

The Offense: The ENEMY generals are the hostess and host wanting to smite you with their swords of warm Italian garlic bread and butter.

The Defense: You. YOU trying to diet in full battle uniform.

The Battle Uniform

Helmet: To protect you from the rain of salty cashews that the ENEMY keeps firing at you from cute little dishes on every coffee table.

Battle Jacket: A trim-fitting Levi denim jacket with pockets to hold your ammunition: .32 caliber celery and raw carrot mortars.

Battle Belt: Metal rings from the tops of diet soda cans for your low-calorie canteen filled with A & W sugar-free root beer. Also five rings to attach your Red Delicious apple grenades. The Battle Belt also holds up your too-big pants from winning all those pitched battles with the ENEMY.

Combat Boots: Special Nike Diet Running Shoes made for Controlled Cheaters. The soles are heavy sponge Romaine lettuce leaves for twisting and turning quickly to avoid the most powerful weapon of the ENEMY: The Goody Table Tank.

The Rifle: YOUR MOUTH. The devastating thirty-two-tooth mint Crest. The most powerful Controlled Cheating weapon in the world that shoots only three bullets: NO THANK YOU.

Easy to carry and can deliver a defensive punch that has never failed to make the ENEMY retreat to their foxholes behind the garbage disposal.

When offered a plate of pepperoni pizza, turn your rifle and shoot oh-so-politely, NO THANK YOU. You will never run out of bullets.

The Enemy Weapon

The Goody Tank Table: An awesome ENEMY war machine that has laid low many a Controlled Cheater. This brutal baby has some of the most powerful guns in the Battle. The Tank fires plates of cheese, cakes, cookies, quiche, and corn bread; bowls of sour cream dip, potato chips, pretzels, and peanuts.

The vicious Goody Tank Table has a secret weapon, too. A human magnet that draws warm Controlled Cheating bodies to it. These poor bodies many times have no control once within the reach of the dreaded Goody Tank.

Never you fret. You are lucky to have that rough-and-ready winner of the Congressional Medal of Slimness, Controlled Cheating combat veteran, ruggedly good-looking with just a touch of gray at the temples, Commander in Chief of All Allied Forces in the Bakery Department of Safeway, Honors graduate of the Dairy Queen Military Academy, and all-around, Baby Ruth chewing, tough son-of-a-gun dieter, "Ike, Omar, Patton, Dutch" Goldberg.

The following are General Goldberg's famous defensive strategies that have been carefully studied by every ENEMY party giver both here and in Arkansas.

The Famous Kitchen Slide: Dieter steps into a Christmas Day dinner, wedding reception, birthday party, or any other Battle and stumbles unsuspecting on the ENEMY'S favorite battleground, The Kitchen.

Quickly move your Combat Boots and slide sideways through the crowd and move directly into the bedroom. Start looking for what your enemy has in the drawers of their night table. NEVER, never do battle in The Kitchen. You're outnumbered.

Mata Hari and Mata Harry: These tricksters are your host and hostess under heavy disguise to lure you into a dangerous high-calorie eating trap.

Some of their favorite ploys are hiding brownies under your salad, cherry pie disguised as broccoli, and lucious, greasy fried chicken molded in the shape of plain yogurt. *Beware!*

Hitting the Beach at Coney Island or C. Day: Soldier, make sure you have your Rifle, Helmet, Battle Jacket, Battle Belt, and Combat Boots when you invade any picnic, barbecue, beach cookout, or any other Battle fought out-of-doors in the fresh air without any cover.

The ENEMY KNOWS that everything tastes better outside, what with homemade potato salad, juicy hot barbecued hamburgers and hot dogs, corn on the cob drenched in two sticks of butter, and all washed down with cold beer and soda. For dessert there's your aunt's chocolate cake with gooey creamy frosting that you have to lick off your hands.

When you hit the beach, dig in and have only *one* burger well done, without the bun, plenty of diet soda, and two bushels of fresh fruit including all the watermelon you can handle.

When the ENEMY sees this, they will turn tail and retreat. You've defeated them again.

Nerve Gas: The sneakiest, dirtiest trick in the ENEMY'S arsenal, Nerve Gas cannot be seen, smelled, or heard. Horribly, it can attack at any large or small party where you don't know a soul and you're trying to find someone to talk to.

Or it can creep up at an Easter Sunday dinner where the Easter Bunny just laid an egg.

Or you're invited to a married couple's small intimate dinner party where they've invited someone "who is just perfect for you."

You guessed it. Nerve Gas causes Nerves and Nervousness, the silent enemy. Twitching hands go into key lime pies and mouths suddenly can open wide enough to accommodate a whole pan of lasagne.

Your only counterattack is to muster your mighty DIET.

Resolve and Nerve

Thus when you're chatting with someone truly wonderful, and you're draped against the bookcase to look as skinny as possible, and the light, witty conversation suddenly drops dead, and your mind turns to oatmeal, I guarantee the awful Nerve Gas will attack.

Drop your hands to your sides and let them dangle. Do not raise them higher than your knees. Square your shoulders and jaw and see if you've got any carrot mortars or apple grenades left. If not, ask the wonderful person to go out on the terrace to watch the submarine races, or into the hall to play with the elevator buttons, or escort them in to see the new shower curtain.

Whatever you do, Soldier, walk, sprint, and run as fast and far as possible from the ENEMY. Get internally tough and think about your Controlled Cheating Day coming up.

Now a word from the Commander In Chief:

"Troops, you will never see V.E. Day, Victory Over Eating. You will never get a ticker-tape parade down Broadway when you return from the Diet Wars. You will never be total victors.

"You will be doing Battle with the ENEMY for the rest of your born days. You will have furloughs on your Controlled Cheating Days, but you will never experience complete victory over fattening foods.

"Take it from this old diet soldier, you will have to fight, gouge, and kick the ENEMY whenever this foul thing rears its ugly head on Non-Cheating Days.

"By now, you are wise, battle-hardened veterans, who can beat back any food challenge.

"Remember, Old Dieters Never Die, They Just Melt Away."

SEVENTY GIMMICKS, TIPS, FUN STUFF, AND OTHER STRANGE PHENOMENA I'VE USED FOR SOCIAL, NON-SOCIAL, AND AWFUL EVENTS

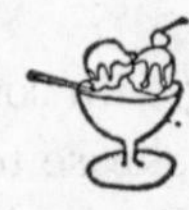

Here's a smorgasbord of stuff I've invented, heard from pals, read about, or eavesdropped on while waiting in line at the corner drug store for the penny scale where I could get my fortune told.

All these one-, two-, three-, four-, or five-liners are laid out on purpose. You have to read them all.

You've probably invented plenty of diet tricks and tips yourself. Drop me a line and let me know yours.

On a Non-Cheating Day, watch other people eat and taste everything with your mind. You get to eat everything and the other guy gets the calories. The biggest problem you'll have with this is drooling in public.

Look for restaurants where you can have Weight Watcher or low-calorie plates.

Order melon, fruit, fish, or tomato juice for appetizers.

Never announce you're on a diet. They'll find out soon enough when they see your slim body.

Mess around with the food on your plate to make it look like you've attacked the food. No sneaky tastes either, when they put on something fattening.

Eat carrots, celery, cauliflower, or fruit at your house before leaving for dinner at a friend's or a restaurant.

At a restaurant, order all vegetables steamed with no butter or sauce.

Trim all visible fat from meat. Use a sharp sword.

On a Controlled Cheating Day, never go into a restaurant or friend's house where at least 50 percent of the people aren't overweight.

When you go to American restaurants, many have a salad bar. Mostly hang around there and be sure and use fresh lemon juice as your dressing.

Always use small plates. Smaller portions always look larger.

Talking, when you're out eating, has less calories than a baked potato with butter and sour cream.

Order plain soups like French onion without the melted cheese, or a clear consommé.

At a big party, where no one is watching, you can diet to your heart's content. Watch out, you can cheat to your heart's content, too.

Never eat "seconds."

Before you order, look at that menu like you're studying for the bar exam.

If it's a Diet Day and you're at a friend's house for dinner, so they won't get upset because you're not eating enough, give them loads of compliments and smack your lips a lot.

Cut your food into small pieces.

Drink a glass of water as soon as you sit down at the table.

Choose dishes low in fats such as huge mixed salads, with fresh lemon dressing, plain baked potato, juices, and vegetables.

Don't pick food off other folks' plates. It's rude unless it's your mother's plate.

At a party, stay as far away as possible from the goody table without ending up on the front lawn or the tree house.

If you get a sandwich, take the top piece of bread off. Then put the two halves with the goodies together. You will have a big fat sandwich and the mustard can run straight down your arm.

Cafeterias are good for dieters. No complete meals. Be sure everything isn't drenched in butter or grease.

On Controlled Cheating Days don't waste calories on dumb cheating foods you don't really want. Become a class junk-food eater.

Going out to a seafood restaurant? Order the fish poached, baked, broiled, boiled, or grilled on a dry grill. Hold the butter and tartar sauce.

Forget fruit cocktails. They're loaded with sugar. Stick to fresh fruit instead.

Eat half of the goodies on your plate if the portions are big enough for a giraffe.

Try a health food or vegetarian eatery. Stay away from the nuts and seeds—too many calories.

Always ask for cottage cheese in place of some fattening food.

When you eat very slooooowly, the taste of the food comes through with vigor.

The twenty potato chips you will slip in your mouth at a party will cost you as many calories as you would spend in two hours normally sitting and shuffling cards.

Remember, you're not a kid anymore. You, Controlled Cheater, don't have to join the "Clean Plate Club!"

In Chinese restaurants, order food with no salt, oil, sugar, or M.S.G. You add a shot of soy sauce when the stuff comes.

Never go anywhere when you're "starving."

Always order diet soda, tomato juice, or one of the fancy waters with a spritz of lime. Only order the water when you're not paying.

Don't pick up your fork until everyone else has begun to eat.

Forget cream sauces, butter sauces, or any sauces through which you can't see the bottom of the bowl.

The roll basket is there for everyone. Don't become a "Diet Bore" by asking the waiter to take it away. You, Controlled Cheater, are not the only one at the table.

Fresh strawberries are a dynamite low-calorie dessert. No sour cream either, sneaky.

Put small portions on your small plate.

If you see a smorgasbord or buffet table in a beanery, party, or pal's home, bolt out the door and head for the hills. Can't do that? Be very, very careful and don't go back for seconds.

The three best, most important words for a dieter, are NO THANK YOU. Maybe you should ink those ten letters on your knuckles.

Order NO complete meals. Get everything separately—as they say in France, a la carte.

The big advantage in Chinese restaurants is that almost everything is cooked to order. So you can get anything you want cooked the way you want it.

Don't eat foods you don't like.

One gimmick I've used for years when I was fat was to help the hostess or host clear the table. I could knock off 5,000 more calories in the kitchen eating mashed potatoes and gravy with my fingers. You just sit there and be rude—and thin.

Be sure you eat tiny bites of everything. No shoveling.

Have the waitress bring salad dressings and all sauces on the side, if you want a little taste. Then you can control how much is sprayed on.

As best you can, keep an empty refrigerator. Only keep what you absolutely must have for your family. I live alone. My fridge looks like I'm about ready to move to Moscow.

Experts say that by 1985 half of the meals we eat will be outside the house. Better learn how to order and nosh in a restaurant.

Portions are huge at a restaurant. Order an extra plate and split with someone else. Saves money, too.

No fried or deep-fried anything.

You can order lobster (big bucks), but you get no butter.

Order foods that require cutting, gnawing, picking, and plenty of horsing around. A good piece of bony chicken or turkey can take forty-five minutes to eat. You'll eat less and make lots of noise.

When ordering, know exactly what you want and do not change, regardless of what the others order.

Eat fresh fruit for dessert.

Eat smoked salmon . . . not the salty kind called lox, as in Goldielox Pizza, a lox-and-onion delight.

Take two bites of everything and throw the rest away.

Order one or two low-calorie appetizers once in a while, instead of one main course.

Eat a plain baked potato, about ninety calories, with no butter or sour cream.

Stay away from cold cuts, luncheon meats, and cheese. They have many hidden calories.

Take the skin off turkey and chicken. This is where the fat hides. You'll save a lot of calories.

If you've got food left on your plate, ask for a Goldberg Bag and take the rest home for another meal.

Pick at your food.

Use your imagination. It's the most important and powerful diet muscle we have.

Forget duck and goose. Very, very fatty fowl. Heavy calories.

Jewish and Italian food can be tricky. Better get a salad with fresh lemon dressing. Unless you can get broiled chicken or fish.

Become a taster instead of an eater at parties, beaneries, and friends' houses.

Finally, one of the best pieces of diet advice I ever got: This one is so hard to do I've been working on it for eleven years with just a little success. You do it too because it's worth the effort:

PUT YOUR FORK OR SPOON DOWN AFTER EVERY BITE. DO NOT PICK IT UP UNTIL AFTER YOU HAVE CHEWED THE FOOD SLOOOOOWLY AND SWALLOWED.

You'll be amazed at how slowly you'll eat and how much more you'll enjoy your goodies.

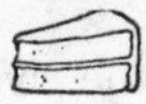

The Last Word: The Thin Evangelist Speaks

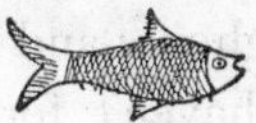

From The Temple of Controlled Cheating
and Heavenly Thinness
Sermon: 11:00 A.M. "Help For The Heavy"

You are fat! Yesiree, brothers and sisters, sisters and brothers, you are obese!

There you sit in the ice box, eating yourselves into oblivion. You're *never* going up to heaven. Do you know why? Because no one can *lift* you, that's why.

Are you tired of being called a nice couple? Are you wearing your old necklace as a wedding ring? Can you be saved? Yes, yes, and amen.

Who will help you lay down that knife and fork? I will, Brother Fats.

Now turn to page forty-three in your Sara Lee hymn book, and we will sing "Shut My Mouth."

"We're gonna leave our bags of candy bars down by the riverside . . . down by the riverside . . . down by the riverside. We're gonna leave our cakes and cookie jars down by the riverside . . . ain't gonna stuff our mouths no more."

(And when we finish our hymns, we say "Amen," not "Pass the Plate.")

Sisters and brothers, I've been fat and I've been skinny. And I'm here to tell you skinny is better. Do I hear a HALLELUJAH.

I haven't forgotten what it's like in the land of dunking doughnuts and peanut brittle.

I haven't forgotten those wild times at the five-stool joints with the great greasy bacon cheeseburgers, pancake houses where warm maple syrup and butter flow out of faucets, and Mexican palaces where the combination platters have enough combined calories to give a computer a hernia.

No, no, no. I haven't forgotten any of that big time eating. How can I forget? I've gone all through the fiery hells of fatness just like you have, sisters and brothers.

Say it with me, now. No more fatness. Louder. NO MORE FATNESS! Can I get a gigantic amen for no more fatness!

I've crawled on my belly, hands, and knees, begging to be taken out in a snowstorm for a dozen hot sticky glazed doughnuts and a quart of cold chocolate milk.

I've screamed up to heaven for a torrential downpour of walnut brownies and vanilla ice cream. Then one day, lying in the gutter filled with fettucini Alfredo, I cried for someone to help me to lose weight and keep it off.

Miracle of miracles, a big strong hand took my shoulder and helped me to my shaky feet. A thundering voice came from I-know-not-where, booming: "You and you alone, Goldberg, are responsible for the way you eat."

Looking around in a heavenly daze, I discovered that the

helping hand and voice came from *me*, from deep inside *my* soul. I deliberated, I meditated, and then it happened.

From the supermarket in my mind came the biggest, best food package of all—Controlled Cheating. The answer from heaven for the desperate dieter. A chock-full-of-wisdom way to lose weight. Now and forever.

THE FIVE COMMANDMENTS OF CONTROLLED CHEATING

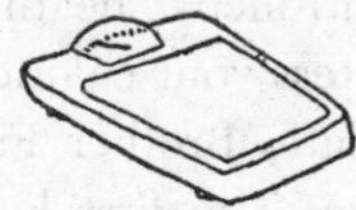

Controlled Cheating is THE answer to losing weight and keeping it off. Dear brothers and sisters, you may rightly ask, how?

1. I know Controlled Cheating works because I am sitting and writing this on a hot Saturday afternoon in early August. For a fat guy who wasn't supposed to be around past the age of thirty, here I am cavorting and playing in my Sperry Topsider canvas shoes, a happy forty-seven years old, and in perfect health (except for one corn, two varicose veins, and one pair of bifocal glasses).

Controlled Cheating works. I lost 175 pounds and have kept it off for twenty-two years. When all else failed in my fat eating life, Cheating Eating rescued me from the hellish depths of hot butterscotch sauce.

2. Controlled Cheating works because it is a program, plan, roadmap, and system. Look at every success, regardless of what, you've had in the world. It had a system. Everything must have a system, a clear individual program that you follow working or

playing. With a good plan, everything you desire and want to accomplish will be possible to achieve.

Haphazard, hit-and-run dieting will never keep your weight off. Besides, it's a hazard. Check the spelling of that word—hap-*hazard!*

3. Controlled Cheating works because you have complete control over everything you eat including the days you are going to cheat and eat. This completely eliminates guilt and depression. And the tremendous burden, of always having to think about what and where you're going to cheat, has disappeared.

Hold on. Hold on. Do I see a repenting brother stumbling off the sawdust trail of Controlled Cheating? Say it, brother. Say what's in your heart. Confess your calories.

"I'm hooked on chocolate, Brother Fats. I can't help myself. My folks never loved me. The first kiss they gave me was a Hershey. From then on, I knew where to find love. But soon plain chocolate wasn't enough. I wanted chocolate-covered raisins, candy bars with almonds! Malteds! Pies! Anything! I can't hold a job. I weigh 300 pounds. My skin's broken out. And to top it all off, my wife ran away. Oh, help me, somebody's got to help me, Brother Fats. What'll I do? What'll I do?"

It's very simple. Stop eating chocolate every day of the week —but one.

(Amazed.) "Gee, I never thought of that. Thank you, brother. Bless you. Just stop eating chocolate six days a week. You're an amazing man, Brother Fats. Stop eating chocolate until the seventh day and then, *bam!* Boy, he's everything they said he was."

Thank you, brother. Chocolate lives!

4. Controlled Cheating works because it makes you laugh and have fun. On your Cheating Eating Days every week, and for two individual vacation weeks every year, you can play and have good things to eat. Plus you learn that *Bozo, Crazy, Uncontrolled Eating Does Not Work!*

5. Controlled Cheating works because every man, woman, child, and golden retriever is going to cheat. Cheating is as natural as the sunrise and is the concrete foundation of the Controlled Cheating Program.

Controlled Cheating is part of our humanness. We all need and deserve a day or days of rest from hard work, especially the brutally hard work of losing weight and keeping it off.

I quote now from The Holy Scriptures, according to the Masoretic Text from The Jewish Publication Society of America, the Book of Genesis, 2:1–3:

"And the heaven and earth were finished, and all the host of them. And on the seventh day God finished His work which He had made; and He rested on the seventh day from all His work which He had made. And God blessed the seventh day, and hallowed it; because that in it He rested from all His work which God in creating had made."

Good luck and Godspeed.